How to Publish in Biomedicine

Biomedicine

500 tips for success

Second Edition

Jane Fraser

Radcliffe Publishing
Oxford • New York

Radcliffe Publishing Ltd
18 Marcham Road
Abingdon
Oxon OX14 1AA
United Kingdom

www.radcliffe-oxford.com
Electronic catalogue and worldwide online ordering facility.

British Library Cataloguing in Publication Data

A catalogue record for this book is available from the British Library.

ISBN-13: 978 1 84619 263 0

Typeset by Advance Typesetting Ltd, Oxon
Printed and bound by TJI Digital, Padstow, Cornwall

Contents

Foreword to the first edition

The Author's Revenge
There was an old editor (your foe),
Who usually preferred to say no,
    He ranted and railed,
    'Till his heart nearly failed,
He died lonely and broken – ho, ho!

Anon, 1823

Such is the miserable life of a journal editor.

First things first. Read this book. It is all true. Beautifully written. Brilliantly argued. You would be a fool to ignore the wise words it has to offer.

If, however, you are pressed for time (and unless you are working at a London teaching hospital, you will be), here is a summary. Structured, of course.

The three A's to acceptance are:

- **Approach**. The covering letter is vital. Editors are showered with manuscripts daily (25 at *The Lancet*). We cannot possibly read through every page of every paper. Nor would we want to. A brief, gently hyperbolic account of what you have done and why it should be irresistible to the editor is a sure way to get noticed. But …
- **Appeal**. I am assuming rejection (which, be honest, is the likely outcome). The editor's decision is *never* final. Editors are jitteringly insecure about their judgements. No one wants to pass up the scientific equivalent of an actor's role in *Jurassic Park*. If your paper has not been peer reviewed, claim tragic injustice and a terrible missed opportunity. If a reviewer's pen has led to editorial refusal, claim undisclosed bias and a poverty of intellect on the part of the advisor. In other words, appeal to the editor's better nature – namely, greed for a higher impact factor.

• **Attitude**. Be quick in your rebuttal of the editor's decision. We have short memories. No recollection of your paper means no chance. And, in all your correspondence, be polite. I have a growing pile of incredibly irate letters from well-known Professors of medicine, all of whom are too used to people saying yes to them. Here is the latest on my desk: 'Although I have not argued the toss with the last three rejections from *The Lancet* of papers in which I have been involved, I think this decision is extremely unfair and certainly I find it very difficult to accept based on the rather meagre contents of your letter. I am becoming increasingly confused about your editorial policy. I really can't accept a rejection ...' (etc, etc). You can imagine that these sort of wails generate billowing gasps of laughter at *The Lancet* and consign the feted Professor's paper to unrecoverable obscurity. Charm, by contrast, works wonders.

Writing is hard, it is true. But when writing is done with others, it can be rewarding – perhaps even pleasurable. Is this not a worthy end in itself, irrespective of the capricious editor?

In all of this publishing palaver, authors should remind themselves that, contrary to their expectations, editors like to be liked. We want to publish your work. So, put your pen down, put your feet up, pour yourself a large vodka, and read on. Even this Foreword was rejected first time around.

Richard Horton
July 1997

About the author

Dr Jane Fraser started her career as a research scientist, but moved into publishing when she realized that 'I liked writing about the experiments more than I liked doing them'. Her long career in biomedical publishing has given her plenty of opportunities both to write herself and to edit the work of scientists and clinicians. She has worked as editorial director of two international medical communications companies and, since 1991, has been a freelance writer and writing-skills trainer. She is also a consulting tutor to the University of Oxford's Continuing Professional Development Centre, where she enjoys helping scientists from many different countries to write more effectively and get their papers published.

More information about open and in-company biomedical writing courses can be obtained from: www.janefraser.com

About this book

Publishing in scientific journals is the true end-product of scientific research. Long after all the presentations are made, and all the details debated, only the publication remains. Studies carried out, but not written up, moulder away in filing cabinets, and are forgotten. Science only exists when it is published in some permanent form, available to all who enquire. At present, that form is usually the peer-reviewed scientific journal.

Today, the pressure on scientists to publish is stronger than ever before. Despite the many complaints about the exploding number of journals and papers, a long list of publications in prestigious journals is taken as a sign of worth. The ability of scientists is judged not only on the quality of their studies, but on the number and quality of their publications. There is a whole science of scoring publications, with the aim of enabling objective decisions about job appointments and grant applications.

Yet, despite the injunction to 'publish and flourish', most scientists have little training in writing papers. A few of us are lucky enough to have a mentor who knows not only how to write, but how to teach. The rest learn to write papers by doing it, and by making mistakes. We waste valuable time submitting papers, only to have them rejected.

Often, these rejections could have been avoided if we had been more thoughtful about where we submitted the paper, or the format we chose. Some rejections are a result of unclear or disorganized writing. While good writing can never compensate for a badly designed study, bad writing can actually obscure good science.

This book is designed to help you get your biomedical papers published. It is based on many years of experience, not only of writing papers, but of teaching scientists from a wide range of backgrounds and many different countries. *They* have taught *me* what scientists really want to know about writing and publishing papers.

There are already plenty of comprehensive textbooks around on scientific writing, but this book is different. It is intended to answer the commonest questions about scientific writing, and to help you avoid the most frequent problems and pitfalls. It is designed to be very practical, and to be used when you are actually writing. You do not have to read it straight through from beginning to end. Just dip into any chapter and you will find a range of tips relevant to the section you are working on right now.

This book is also very realistic, in that it recognizes that you may not have very much time for writing. So it includes chapters on managing your time for writing and revising, overcoming writer's block and using technology to make your writing more efficient.

I hope that everyone who reads this book will find useful hints that they can use again and again to help ease the process of writing and publishing papers. There is no reason why this process should always be long and painful. As with all other walks of life, when you know what you are trying to achieve, you will be able to use the skills you already have to maximize your potential. You might even have time to do some research. Good luck!

Jane Fraser
January 2008

Acknowledgements

The book grew out of the questions and suggestions of participants in all the courses I have taught on scientific writing and publishing. Special thanks are therefore due to the Continuing Professional Development Centre and Department of Medical Sciences at the University of Oxford for providing the platform for many of these courses. I am also indebted to the Joint Research Centres of the European Union, to the European Molecular Biology Laboratory, to Gothenburg University and to the Flanders Institute of Biotechnology. Thanks are also due to the many publishing and pharmaceutical companies and their staff who have kindly invited me to teach courses.

Sincere thanks also go to Liz Wager for her many helpful suggestions on the manuscript of the first edition. Finally, I would also like to express my gratitude to the countless friends and colleagues who have contributed over the years to my store of tips. Without them, this book could not have been written.

1

What do you want to write?

If you want to publish something in a biomedical journal or magazine, you will need to decide on the right format for what you have to say. This section defines some of the commonest types of publication, to help you decide into which category your publication fits.

Use these definitions in conjunction with the advice on choosing a journal in Chapter 4. The important thing is to choose the right format for the information you wish to convey, and to send your paper to a journal or magazine that accepts that format.

▲ Describe an experimental or observational study in an original research paper ...

Full-length original research papers are the main category of paper included in any peer-reviewed journal. Think, however, about whether your paper might have a better chance of publication as a short communication (see below). Chapters 5–9 give more advice on how to prepare an original research paper.

▲ ... Or a 'short communication'

Some journals also publish 'short communications' or 'brief communications'. These are abbreviated descriptions of original research studies, with a strict limitation on the number of words or pages allowed (see Chapter 4).

▲ Describe an unusual case in a case report

Only some journals accept case reports – descriptions of one or more patients that illustrate some novel clinical problem or its solution. Be sure that your case history is really as interesting as you think it is – it will have to tell a story that has not been told before. Case reports are most likely to be published if they describe:

- a previously unknown disease or syndrome (it still happens occasionally)
- a previously unsuspected causal association between two diseases
- a new and unexpected variation in the usual pattern of a disease
- a hitherto unreported adverse drug reaction or interaction.

▲ Use a letter to the editor to give a brief description of a study …

One way of publishing data that would not make a full-length paper is as a letter to the editor in a journal that accepts this format. Some journals have a separate section for 'research letters'. Keep your letter brief and to the point. When describing original research in a letter, you can usually include a couple of references, but no figures or tables. Note that if you publish something as a letter to the editor you will not be able to publish the same study again as a full paper. Bear in mind also that only a few letters ever get indexed in PubMed, so although your letter will be citeable as a research publication, it will be less likely to be identified and read than a full paper.

▲ … Or to comment on other studies the journal has recently published

You may wish to comment on a study recently published in the journal, and amplify the comment with a few lines reporting your own findings, e.g. 'In their recent paper (*Elderly Issues* 2007; **36**: 2–7), Smith and Brown reported that gerontazole is an effective treatment for Portillo's disease in elderly patients. In our own pilot study in six women aged 95 years or older, we found that …'

▲ … Or simply to state your point of view on a topical issue

Lastly, the letter to the editor can simply give your opinion or state some relevant facts on any topical issue. For a young scientist, having a letter published in a top journal can be a useful career boost. The chief criterion for acceptance of this kind of letter is that it should be of interest to the journal's readers. Make sure that, in commenting on someone else's research or practice, you do not inadvertently say anything that could be construed as libellous – keep it as impersonal as possible. Make it clear in the letter that you give your permission to publish (some letters are written for the eyes of the editor only).

▲ Write a review article to summarize the literature or a series of studies

Only some journals accept review articles. They are often commissioned by the editor, so a review article submitted with no prior notice may be courting rejection. However, editors of journals that publish review articles are always open to new ideas, so contact them first to see if your suggested topic is welcome. For more about review articles, see Chapter 20.

▲ Write an editorial to put forward a new or controversial point of view

Look closely, and you will see that 'editorials' and similar articles are not always written by the editor of the journal, but also by invited contributors, well-known and well-respected in their field. You are unlikely to get an editorial accepted if it is submitted speculatively. However, if you have something really important to say, it is worth approaching the editor to see if they would consider inviting you to write an editorial.

▲ Write an informal article to reach a wider audience, to describe recent events or to tell a personal story

You may find that not everything you want to say fits into the categories described above. A few journals include informal articles alongside peer-reviewed research papers. These 'news-and-views' articles do not carry the academic kudos of a peer-reviewed paper, but they can still help attract attention to you and your institution. They can also be fun to write. For example, you might want to write about something 'newsy' like 'How our geriatric unit cut antibiotic costs' or 'The Global Congress of Gastroenterology 2007: a surgeon's view'. You might also want to write something more personal, or even humorous – 'Medicine at 30 000 feet'.

Opportunities for informal writing may also be available in magazines and newsletters for your fellow professionals or the general public. For example, you might have a suitable idea for the *New Scientist, Scientific American* or *Trends in Pharmaceutical Sciences*. If you are unsure whether the article you have in mind would be appropriate, you can contact the editor for advice. Advice on writing informal scientific and medical articles is given in Chapter 23.

2

Understanding the publishing process

If you do any kind of biomedical research, you are going to become very familiar with the process of publishing scientific papers. For better or worse, the success of your research career will depend on your ability to get your research published in *peer-reviewed* journals. So, it pays to be familiar with the process and the people involved.

▲ Familiarize yourself with the publishing process

Figure 2.1 outlines the typical progress of a paper from submission to publication. You submit your paper to the editor. Often, the editor will perform a preliminary screen on all papers that are submitted to the journal, before sending 'possibles' out for peer review. The editor then makes the decision to accept or reject your paper, on the advice of the reviewers (referees). Usually, you will have to make some amendments, taking into advice the reviewers' comments. Once your paper is accepted, it will be edited to conform with journal style, and proofs returned to you for correction. Only then will it finally be ready for publication.

▲ Understand the roles of the people involved

At different stages of the publication process, you may find yourself dealing with:

- the editor
- reviewers (also known as referees)
- the managing editor
- copy-editors (also known as sub-editors or desk editors).

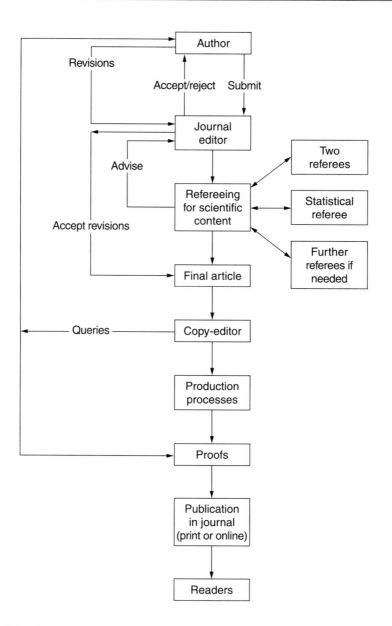

Figure 2.1 The publishing process – a simplified view.

Each has a specific role to play in publishing the journal. Let's look at their roles one by one.

▲ The editor decides whether to accept or reject papers

The editor of a peer-reviewed journal is always an eminent scientist with many years of experience. The biggest and most prestigious journals often have full-time editors – for example, the editors of *The Lancet*, *New England Journal of Medicine* and *Nature* are paid professionals, with a distinguished academic career behind them. However, the editors of smaller, specialized journals are almost always part-time and unpaid, fitting in their editorial role alongside the demands of research, teaching and clinical responsibilities. The editor is usually advised by an editorial board of other eminent scientists or clinicians, who may sometimes also act as reviewers (see below).

▲ The reviewers advise the editor

Reviewers may be members of the editorial board, personal contacts of the editor, or simply chosen from a database of suitably qualified people. Editors are constantly adding to the pool of reviewers. Sometimes, they will remove from the pool those who do not provide reviews on time, or do not meet the journal's standards for scientific stringency and attention to detail. The details of the peer-review process vary slightly between journals, but the general principle remains the same. Typically, the editor will send out copies of the paper to two reviewers simultaneously. Others may use a single reviewer to screen the paper, followed by a second reviewer if the paper is deemed worthy of further consideration. A third reviewer may be called in if the first two disagree, as sometimes happens. Many journals also now send papers out for a separate statistical review – in fact, statistical inadequacy is one of the commonest reasons for rejection. The reviewers do not actually make the decision to accept or reject the paper – they merely advise the editor.

▲ The managing editor oversees the day-to-day running of the journal

Most larger journals employ a managing editor to oversee the day-to-day running of the journal and supervise the work of the copy-editors (see below). The managing editor is often the easiest person to contact if you have questions about non-scientific matters (for example, a request for a copy of the Instructions to Authors, or a query about when your paper is to be published). However, queries regarding the scientific content of your paper must always be addressed to the editor.

▲ Copy-editors (also known as sub-editors or desk editors) edit your paper to journal style

Once a paper has been accepted for publication it will go through a process known as copy-editing. Most journals employ copy-editors. The copy-editor will make small changes to the paper so that it conforms exactly to the journal's 'house style'. The house style lays down rules on everything from the size of headings to the abbreviations allowed to the formatting of references. The copy-editor will also correct grammatical and spelling errors, improve poorly constructed sentences and paragraphs and generally polish the manuscript to publication standard.

▲ Remember that credibility depends on peer review

In peer-reviewed journals, original research papers or review articles are only published if they meet the standards set by one or more independent expert reviewers. Publication in peer-reviewed journals means that your work has been given a 'seal of approval' by the scientific community.

▲ Peer review acts as 'quality control' for the scientific content of papers

Readers will assume that peer-reviewed papers have been checked for:

- a logical starting hypothesis, in the light of existing knowledge
- appropriate experimental design and statistical analysis
- complete and precise description according to a standard scientific format
- reasonable conclusions supported by your own experiments and those of others.

▲ Peer review has its limitations

Of course, publication in a peer-reviewed journal is no guarantee that the conclusions drawn in a paper are the ultimate answer to any particular scientific question. Biomedical research is not like that – it deals in probabilities rather than absolute proofs. Even papers by the most respected scientists are regularly revealed to have been 'wrong' in the light of further research. What's more, the peer review process is undoubtedly imperfect – it can be cumbersome, time-consuming and open to bias. However, it is the best method so far devised for 'quality control' in science.

▲ Remember that reviewers are very busy people

Reviewers give many hours of service to scientific journals – usually completely free of charge. Without their goodwill the whole system would collapse. Most scientists feel it to be their duty to their fellow researchers to take part in the peer-review process. Most say that they find it interesting and educational. However, because the best reviewers are constantly in demand, the time they can devote to reading and commenting on each paper is limited. So, it pays to make sure that your paper is written clearly and concisely, so that the reviewer can make a swift evaluation of the scientific content without having to struggle with impenetrable writing.

▲ Expect your paper to be 'blinded' when it is sent to the reviewers …

In order to make the reviewing process more fair, many journals adopt a policy of 'blinding' – the authors' names are taken off the paper so that the reviewer does not know where the paper comes from and can therefore make an unbiased assessment of its merits. In the same way, the reviewers' names are usually not included on the list of comments sent to authors (so that the reviewers can be as frank as they like without fear of complaint).

▲ … But do not expect always to be assured anonymity

Of course, blinding can never be controlled completely – it may be obvious to the reviewer from the text and references which research group carried out the study. In a specialized area of research, where everyone knows everyone else, the data may already have been discussed at conferences and informal meetings, and both reviewer and author will be able to make an informed guess about each other's identity. Authors may also know the identity of one of the reviewers if they actually suggested them to the editor. With these problems in mind, some journals are now using a system of 'open' review, or asking reviewers whether they are willing to have their names revealed to authors.

▲ Normally, you will not have to pay to have your paper published ...

Traditional peer-reviewed journals cover their expenses by selling subscriptions and advertising. In the case of society journals, the journal is at least partially funded by membership fees. Authors are not normally charged for the publication of their papers.

▲ ... except in some online journals

A new model is emerging among online-only journals, which cannot raise enough funds through subscriptions or advertising to cover their costs. Authors are asked to pay a substantial fee to cover the costs of publication, though papers are still peer-reviewed. Fees are waived for authors from developing countries.

▲ ... and under certain specific circumstances

Other exceptions to the 'no payment' rule are:

- some journals may ask you to pay for the reproduction of photographs (particularly colour photographs), which are expensive to print
- a few journals publish short papers free, but expect authors to pay a 'page rate' for papers over a certain length. This is not the same as being a 'pay journal' (see below)
- there are a small number of 'pay journals' that require the author to pay for publication. Some of these operate a system of peer review, others do not. In general, they are considered to be of lower status than the standard type of peer-reviewed journal.
- some journals charge an optional fee for immediate online open access. This means that readers can obtain your paper free of charge as soon as it is published, instead of having to pay for a pdf according to the journal's usual policy.

▲ Be prepared to make revisions

Once the reviewers have commented on the paper, the editor will write telling you the fate of your paper. You may be told that it:

- has been rejected outright
- has been accepted (usually subject to at least minor revisions)
- has been rejected, but may be reconsidered if various revisions can be made.

It is very unusual for a paper to be accepted exactly as it stands. Reviewers are normally asked to provide detailed comments, either to help the author understand the reasons for rejection or to explain the revisions required. Some reviewers are more helpful than others in explaining what changes will make the paper 'publishable'.

▲ Do not expect the publishing process to be fast

The publishing process can be extremely lengthy. A wait of six months to a year from submission to publication is typical – some journals may take longer. This is not surprising when you consider that the peer-review process may take three or four months, and the journal's editing and production processes another three or four months. Some journals do not appear very often, so there may also be a backlog of accepted papers waiting to be published. For advice on how to speed up the publishing process, see Chapter 4. Online-only journals, which do not have to go through print production processes, are often faster than traditional journals.

▲ Be prepared to answer the copy-editor's queries promptly and courteously

The copy-editor does not criticize the scientific content of a manuscript, but will try to pick up any ambiguities or inconsistencies – for example, if the numbers given in a table and those given in the text do not match exactly. After editing your paper, the copy-editor will often submit a list of queries for your attention. If these queries sometimes seem niggling, remember that the copy-editor is there to help you – by detecting errors, however trivial, they protect the journal's reputation for accuracy, saving you from potential embarrassment.

▲ It is your responsibility to check proofs carefully

After your manuscript has been copy-edited, it will be typeset and page proofs returned to you for approval. This will be the last chance you have to see your paper before it is published, so you will have to read the proofs carefully. It is *your* responsibility to ensure that there are no errors, so be sure to check crucial elements like numbers especially carefully. You must return the proofs on time to ensure that you do not forfeit your place in the queue for publication.

3

Original research – what can be published?

The importance of publication as a measure of career success leads many scientists to try to publish as much as possible. On the other hand, editors and other publishing pundits constantly complain that readers are being overwhelmed by too many papers. Here are some tips about what is permissible, and what is not. For more information, see the Uniform Requirements for Manuscripts Submitted to Biomedical Journals www.icmje.org.

▲ Generally speaking, you cannot publish the same data twice

Journals are very strict about 'repetitive' or 'multiple' publication. This means that you cannot publish the same data twice. When you submit your paper, you will normally be expected to confirm that the content of your paper has not been published elsewhere.

▲ An exception *may* be made for papers previously published in another language

If your paper was previously published in another language, a translated 'secondary' version may be accepted by another journal, provided that:

- the editors of both journals are kept fully informed
- the papers are published at least two weeks apart
- the secondary version faithfully reflects the data and interpretation of the original (i.e. is a translation rather than a rewrite)

- the secondary version is written for a different group of readers
- the secondary version informs the audience of that fact and gives a reference to the original.

▲ Publication of an abstract or poster does not count as prior publication …

You can publish your data as an abstract or poster at a conference without pre-judicing publication in a journal. Note that when you do publish your study in a journal, you may add data or change your analysis or interpretation; this is perfectly acceptable. You can usually present the same data at more than one meeting. However, a few large meetings stipulate that the data should not have been previously presented at another meeting.

▲ … Nor does an oral conference presentation

Oral presentation of your data at a conference does not count as prior publication. Nor does a report of your presentation in a newspaper, unless it contains additional data, tables or illustrations. You should, however, be cautious about giving press interviews before you have published your study (see below).

▲ Do not pre-empt publication by releasing data to the press

There have been cases where information from a study that had been accepted but not yet published was released to the popular media. This is a violation of the policies of many journals. Very occasionally, early release of data may be acceptable – for example, to warn the public of health hazards. In this case, the release of data must be negotiated with the editor of the journal in question.

▲ Do not try to slice your data too thinly

'Salami publication' or 'divided publication' are terms sometimes used to describe studies that are sliced very thinly in order to obtain several publications from the same data set. Sometimes, this seems justifiable. For example, some very large studies contain so much data they take years to analyse. The full story could fill a book. It is surely reasonable to publish such studies in segments. Other examples are more debatable. For example, there is a tendency for individual centres involved in large, multicentre trials to want to publish their own data, especially if they foresee a long wait until the whole study is published. However, many leading clinical journals have said that they disapprove of this practice, and that it could jeopardize the final (full) publication.

4

Selecting the
right journal

The first rule of successful publication is to *send your paper to the right journal*. However good the science is, however well written the paper, it can fail at the first hurdle if it is sent to the wrong place. So let us take a look at how you select the right journal for your paper.

▲ Draw up a shortlist of possible journals in order of preference

You can save yourself time and trouble if you know where you are submitting your paper before you begin to write. So think about this early – even before you complete the research. Then you can do a little homework to make sure that you are sending your paper to an appropriate journal.

▲ Think carefully about who will want to read your paper

The whole point of scientific publishing is to communicate your research to the right audience. So start by thinking about who you want to read your paper. For example, if it is a medical paper of interest to doctors in a wide range of specialties, you may want to choose a general clinical journal. On the other hand, if you are conducting superspecialized research that is of interest to only a few hundred scientists worldwide, you may want to choose a superspecialized journal that is read only by those people. Most papers will come somewhere in the middle, and will find a place in journals that cover a broad area such as neuroscience, genetics or cardiology.

▲ Ask your colleagues for advice

Your fellow researchers will be able to tell you about their experiences with different journals – which ones they think are most prestigious, which are most difficult to get into, which publish fastest, and so on. You could also ask your librarian for his or her opinion on which journals are the 'best' and most frequently used.

▲ Look first at the journals you read yourself

The first journals to consider are those that you and your colleagues read regularly. If you look in these journals to find the studies that interest *you*, your own study is likely to fit in well with the journal's policies and preferences. In some areas of research the right journal will be obvious. If you are working in a very specialized field there may be only a handful of specialist journals to which you would consider sending your manuscript.

▲ Check whether your learned society publishes a journal

Check out the scientific societies to which you and your colleagues belong. If your society publishes a journal, the chances are that your paper will fit into their preferred spectrum of subjects.

▲ Review the literature to see where similar papers are published

If you are new to a field, or if your research does not fit neatly into any journal with which you are familiar, you can still check where papers on a similar topic have been published. You will almost certainly have done a computer search to look for relevant references, so check which journals come up time and time again on your reference list – they can be assumed to be receptive to your particular topic.

▲ Consider *all* the journals whose readers might be interested in your work

There is no need to be confined to your own narrow field. For example, as a geneticist, you might be most familiar with genetics journals, but your paper on the genetics of cystic fibrosis might find a wider readership in a clinical journal such as *Lung*.

▲ Remember that a full-length, original research paper may not be your only option

If you have conducted a piece of original research, you will probably want to report it in a full scientific paper with abstract, introduction, methods, results, discussion and conclusions. Not everything published in scientific journals is a full, formal research paper, however. Many journals also publish 'short communications' (a sort of mini-paper), case reports and letters to the editor (see Chapter 1).

▲ Check that the journal accepts papers in the format you have chosen

Look at a complete copy of the journal for guidance. If the answer to your query is not obvious from the journal's website, you can simply email them to ask 'Do you have a format for short communications?' or 'Do you accept case reports?'

▲ Using the 'short communication' format may increase your chances of acceptance

It is quite common for journals to send back a full paper and suggest that it be rewritten as a short communication – so think about whether it should be written as a short communication in the first instance! The short communication format is particularly appropriate for small studies, pilot studies, or studies using standard methodology that need not be described in great detail. Using the short communication format may increase your chances of acceptance and/or rapid publication (see below).

▲ Put your shortlist of journals in rank order, from first choice to last choice

All journals are not equal. Some are acknowledged leaders, while others are middle of the field and some also-rans. Everyone would like to have their research published in the 'top' journals, as this implies that it is of the best quality. You will probably already have formed an idea of which journals are the 'best' in your field. If not, ask your colleagues for their opinions, If you are still not sure, look at where the most important and influential papers in your field have been published in the last few years. Although seminal work does sometimes appear for the first time in little-known journals, world opinion leaders usually publish their work in the 'best' journals.

▲ For a quantitative measure of a journal's status, look at the impact factor

'League tables' are published for scientific journals by Journal Citation Reports® (Thomson Scientific). The best known of the various measures they use is the 'impact factor'. This is the number of times articles from the journal were cited in the previous two years. This gives an indication of how many people read articles in the journal, and how important they think they are. Impact factors can be used to compare journals, but only within the same scientific field, as they are influenced by the popularity of the subject matter as well as the quality of the journal. Nowadays academic institutions attach considerable importance to whether job or grant applicants have published papers in journals with high impact factors. Your librarian will be able to give you further information, or contact: http://scientific.thomson.com/products/jcr

▲ Think carefully about whether your paper is really likely to be accepted by the top journals in your field

No reputable peer-review journal accepts every paper it receives, but there are wide differences in journals' rejection rates. Leading journals such as the *New England Journal of Medicine (NEJM)* accept as few as 10% of the papers that are submitted to them. The *NEJM*'s criteria for acceptance are tough – not only does the science have to be excellent but the findings have to have the potential to change clinical practice. Other top journals are similarly demanding.

▲ Consider the implications of rejection from a top journal

You may feel that your paper is of the highest quality and that it is worth trying to get it published in, say, *Nature*, *The Lancet*, the *Journal of the American Medical Association* (*JAMA*) or the *NEJM*. The worst that can happen is a delay while your paper is considered, during which time you cannot send it anywhere else. Publication in such a journal will certainly be a feather in your cap. On the other hand, you may prefer to lower your sights just a little and send your paper to a specialist, but still prestigious, journal where it will have a better chance of acceptance – say 40%. Or you may decide that you would rather minimize your risk of rejection and send your paper to a less demanding journal where you have a higher chance of acceptance – say 80%. Some online journals have a policy of accepting all papers that meet their minimum quality standards – a policy sometimes called 'bias-to-publish'.

▲ Remember that most journals will happily tell you their rejection/acceptance rates

How do you know what a journal's acceptance/rejection rate is? Well, you can ask them – some will be quite happy to give you that information. If not, you can usually get an adequate idea from the prestige of the journal (see above) and the experiences of any of your colleagues who have submitted papers to the same journal.

▲ If you are eager to reach a large number of readers, look at the journal's circulation

It may be important to you that your paper reaches a large number of readers. On the other hand, you may not care too much as long as the *right* few hundred people get to know about your findings. If you are interested, the advertising department of your chosen journal will usually be able to tell you about the circulation of the journal (how many copies are sold). They may also be able to give you a breakdown of the readership by specialty and by country – they produce these statistics to help them sell space to advertisers. By law, US journals print their circulation in the journal. The highest circulation journals are usually the leading general clinical journals and the journals of large societies.

▲ Find out how fast your paper is likely to be published

Journals vary widely in the time taken from submission of a paper to its eventual publication. Speed of publication can be affected by:

• how fast the editor and reviewers get round to looking at papers. Some journals set strict time-limits for review while others are more relaxed

- how often the journal is published. Generally speaking, your paper will take longer to come out in a journal that is only published twice a year than in one that is published every month
- whether the journal has a large backlog of papers waiting to be published. Journals vary in how many accepted papers they have queuing up for publication.

Most journals will happily give you an estimate of the average time from submission to publication (or at least from acceptance to publication), though few will offer any guarantees.

▲ Choose your journal carefully if you want fast publication

There may be certain circumstances in which rapid publication is important to you. For example, in an extremely competitive field of research, you may want the kudos of being published before a rival group (no-one said that science was entirely fair and objective). If this is the case, the four strategies described below may help (though none are guaranteed to work).

▲ Rapid publication strategy 1: Submit your paper to a prestigious weekly journal

Being published frequently, journals like *Nature* or *The Lancet* tend to have short lead-times and will usually let you have an accept/reject decision quickly. On the other hand, they reject most of the papers submitted to them. You will have to decide if your study is interesting enough and of sufficiently good quality to stand a chance of being seriously considered, let alone accepted.

▲ Rapid publication strategy 2: Try a journal that specializes in rapid publication

Online-only journals often have short submission-to-publication times. Some printed journals also specialize in rapid publication.

▲ Rapid publication strategy 3: Keep it short

Editors usually have a specific number of pages to fill every month. So a compact three-page paper *may* stand more chance of finding an empty slot than a 15-page monster. Some journals actually include a short communication format; others simply have a mix of shorter and longer papers. There is no reason why you should not enquire whether shorter papers are likely to be published more rapidly. However, do not expect any guarantees, especially before the editor has even seen the paper.

▲ Rapid publication strategy 4: Ask to have your paper fast-tracked

If the topic is of critical scientific importance, or has implications for public health or safety, remember that some journals have a system for fast-tracking papers.

▲ Discuss your choice with your co-authors

If your paper is to have more than one author, make sure that all co-authors agree on which journal is to be your first choice, and on the fall-back options in case of rejection. If there are any differences of opinion, it is important to resolve them as early as possible, so that you can write the paper to meet the requirements of the target journal.

5

Planning your writing

Just as careful planning underlies all good research projects, it is also essential to good scientific writing. When reviewers complain that something is badly written, often what they mean is that it is badly organized. Without good organization it is impossible to write clearly or concisely. This section will help you to plan your writing for greater clarity and readability.

▲ Planning is essential, especially in large documents

Careful planning is especially important with longer pieces of writing, such as a thesis, a review article or a book. It is also crucial in the discussion and introduction sections of original research papers. Without good organization, readers and reviewers will be unable to follow the logic of your argument, and may underestimate the importance of your paper.

▲ Take time to plan

If you have a deadline looming, you may feel under pressure to start writing. But try not to be tempted to jump right in without planning your writing first. Time invested at this stage is well worthwhile – it will save you time later. The proportion of your writing time that should be spent in planning will naturally vary with the type of project and your personal working habits, but could be as much as a third of your total writing time.

▲ Organize your writing to help your readers

Readers expect to see a logical flow in any piece of writing. If no structure is imposed by the writer, the reader will be confused. When writing a scientific document, you should aim to do all the sorting and classifying of information for your readers. You need to provide them with a route map through your paper. Think carefully about your readers' needs and how you can organize your writing to meet those needs.

▲ Remember to plan at different levels within your document

You need to plan and organize within:

- the document as a whole (although the main sections of an original research paper are already dictated by the IMRAD format – introduction, methods, results and discussion)
- the main sections
- subsections dealing with different ideas or arguments
- paragraphs
- sentences.

▲ Try mind-mapping

Mind-mapping is a technique developed by psychologist Tony Buzan. It is based on the idea that people do not naturally think in rigid hierarchies or lists. Instead, the human mind darts around from subject to subject, moving naturally and creatively from one topic to another, 'growing' one idea from another. Mind-mapping is a way of capturing this 'radiant thinking' in a visual form, which can then be used to develop a more rigid structure. Figure 5.1 shows a mind map for a review article. I used mind-mapping when writing this book, and find it a very useful technique. Books on mind-mapping and mind-mapping software are listed in Chapters 31 and 33. Note that some mind-mapping software allows you to add text notes to branches, and then export the whole thing to a Word file, thus providing a quick way of generating a first draft.

▲ Try the 'yellow sticky' note technique for organizing ideas ...

Another way of making sense of a large number of ideas is to jot and key topics in note form on 'yellow sticky' Post-it™ notes. You can then lay these out on your desk – or even the wall or floor – and move them around until an appropriate plan emerges. You can combine this technique very effectively with mind-mapping (see above).

▲ ... And their associated references

Another way of using the 'yellow sticky' approach is to write one Post-it note for each reference, noting the author and title of the reference and the key points you

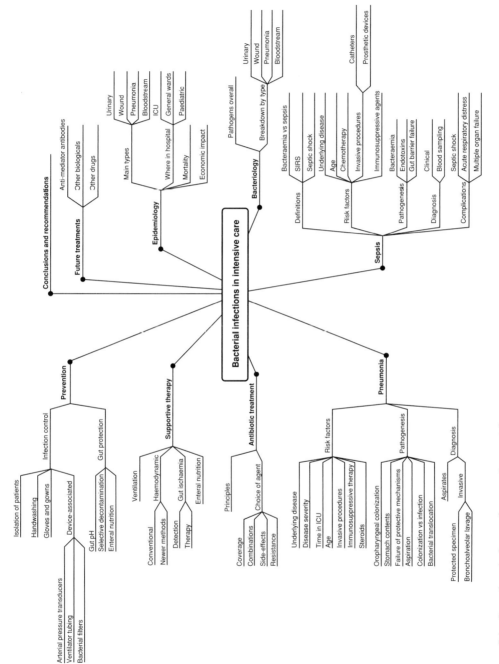

Figure 5.1 Sample mind-map for a review article.

want to extract from it. You can then move these around as before – a great way of planning introductions, discussions and whole review articles (see Chapters 9, 15 and 20).

▲ Try building pyramids of ideas

A pyramid consists of a single brick at the top (the 'big idea' of the article). Under this are several bigger bricks (supporting facts or ideas), and under these still more smaller bricks (smaller facts or ideas). Make sure that you introduce the big bricks first, before going on to support them with the smaller bricks. Never have piles of little bricks lying around with no discernible structure.

▲ Try using the outline function on your word processor

Most well-known word-processing programs, including Word and WordPerfect, have an outline function that will allow you to organize your ideas as a hierarchy of headings. An outline of this kind will help you to define your main sections, subsections and sub-subsections. However, it is often best to precede this phase of planning with a more open phase such as mind-mapping, to make sure you do not get stuck in the rut of straight-line thinking.

▲ Set yourself a word or page budget

A word or page budget is a plan allocating a certain number of words or pages for the whole document and for each section within it. Setting such a budget will help you to:

• avoid wasting time by writing more than you need
• assign the right amount of text to each section.

If you have ever written a 1000-word introduction to a 2000-word paper, or tried to cut your thesis from 60 000 words to meet a statutory limit of 50 000 words, you will understand why a word or page budget is necessary.

▲ Do not forget the journal may have length limits

Many journals will lay down limits in the instructions to authors not only for the maximum length of different kinds of paper (pages or words), but also for the numbers of tables and figures. Check these limits before you start to write your paper.

▲ Organize at the micro- as well as at the macro-level

Meticulous planning will allow you to organize your writing in advance, as far as the paragraph level if you like. However, at least some of your organization will have to be done as you write – or rather, as you edit what you have written. Chapters 24 and 26 tell you more about how to organize your sentences and paragraphs.

▲ Follow guidelines for structuring clinical papers

Note that many clinical medical journals now require that randomized controlled trials be reported according to the Consolidated Standards of Reporting Trials (CONSORT Statement; www.consort-statement.org). Separate guidelines are available on the same website for systematic reviews and meta-analyses (QUORUM), meta-analyses of observational studies (MOOSE), studies of diagnostic accuracy (STARD), and reporting of observational studies (STROBE).

▲ Check whether your chosen journal supplies a template

Some journals supply an electronic template to help you format your paper correctly into the right sections. Templates for selected journals are also available in some reference management programs.

6

Research papers and reviews: titles

Some people might say that the title is the most important part of a paper. After all, how do *you* decide which papers to read? Probably by scanning down a journal's title page or a list of titles downloaded from an online database. So it pays to think carefully about the title of your paper and how you can use it to attract readers.

▲ Get the length right

As always, consult the Instructions to Authors, issued by the publisher. Many journals are quite specific about the length of titles and their format. Length may be specified in number of lines, number of words, or even in number of characters. If in doubt, limit the title to not more than two lines of printed text.

▲ Get the format right

The Instructions to Authors may contain rules about how they would like the title to be written. If in doubt, look at the journal for examples of its usual style. For example, some journals specify that the title should consist of a single sentence; others allow subtitles. Still others allow colons or dashes to join two parts of the title. Some like the use of questions in the title; others do not. The *NEJM* does not like titles in the 'declarative' format (see below), while others are quite happy to accept this style.

▲ Make the title reader friendly

Make sure that the title contains all the information that you would like when deciding whether or not to read a paper. Think about what would be relevant to your readers. Thus, for an original paper, 'Efficacy of grottomycin and scabicillin in sinusitis in adults' would be better than 'Antibiotic treatment of upper respiratory tract infections'. Titles that are too general can be misleading.

▲ Include the keywords that readers will be searching for

Think about which words your target readers will be looking for when deciding whether or not to read an article and remember all the people who conduct a titles-only search as a way of narrowing down the number of items retrieved by on-line searching. That is why it would be important to have 'grottomycin and scabicillin' in the title, instead of something vague like 'macrolides and penicillins'.

▲ Include all key information

As E J Huth says in *Medical Style and Format*, 'The title should be as informative of the article's content as possible within a reasonable length'. So, in an original research paper, it is helpful to your readers to include, where relevant, information on:

• independent and dependent variables involved
• the species, subjects or patient group studied
• condition of animals/subjects/patients
• the experimental approach.

Thus, it would be even more helpful to readers to add key experimental details to the title of the antibiotic study: 'Efficacy of grottomycin and scabicillin in sinusitis in adults: a double-blind trial'. If your chosen journal dislikes the 'title : subtitle' format you could try 'A double-blind comparison of the efficacy of grottomycin and scabicillin in sinusitis in adults'. However, this would have the defect of leaving the keywords until late in the title (see below).

▲ Make sure the most important keywords are near the beginning of the title

Readers' concentration tends to be highest towards the beginning of a sentence, so it will help to attract their attention if you put the most important word or words near the beginning. For example, readers are more likely to be looking for the names of the antibiotics 'grottomycin' and 'scabicillin' than they are for 'double-blind trial'. Even though the experimental detail is relevant and useful, in this example it would be more reader friendly to leave it until last.

▲ If the journal allows it, consider giving the conclusion in the title

Some journals will encourage you to use declarative titles – that is, titles that give the key result of the study, e.g. 'Grottomycin is more effective than scabicillin in sinusitis in adults'. Declarative titles can be helpful to readers when you have a single, strong, clear conclusion. However, some journals, such as the *NEJM*, prefer indicative titles – titles that state what the study is about, but stop short of giving the key conclusion. Their argument is that it is up to the readers to decide whether the conclusion is justified on the basis of the results presented.

▲ If you do state the conclusion in the title, think carefully about how 'aggressive' it sounds

Titles worded in the active voice, such as 'Metoprolol inhibits progression of athero-sclerosis in cholesterol-fed rabbits', sound 'stronger' than those worded in the passive voice, such as 'Inhibition of progression of atherosclerosis by metoprolol in cholesterol-fed rabbits'. It all depends on whether you want the tone to be vigorous and challenging or mild and restrained.

▲ Avoid wasting words

Phrases like 'in the treatment of', 'studies on', 'report of a case of' can often be omitted with no loss of meaning. Readers will exercise their common sense. Often, depending on the style of the journal, you can use a more 'telegraphic' style, getting rid of words such as 'the' and 'a'.

▲ For CONSORT papers, consider putting 'randomized' in the title

The CONSORT guidelines for reporting clinical trials state that the allocation of participants to interventions should be mentioned in the title or abstract. In practice, this often means putting it in the title, e.g. *Efficacy and safety of grottomycin versus scabicillin in sinusitis in adults: a randomized double-blind trial.*

▲ Avoid abbreviations in titles

Abbreviations could lead to the paper being missed in on-line searches, and may be confusing to readers unfamiliar with the subject. Most journals will not allow any abbreviations in the title (apart from the abbreviations for SI units).

▲ Do not forget your running title

The running title (sometimes called a running head) is a short phrase that appears at the top or bottom of every page or every other page. It is designed to help readers find their way around the journal, so that if they open it in the middle of a paper they know what it is about. A running title is usually requested in the journal's Instructions to Authors, and is usually given on the title page. It should be recognizable as a short version of the title, focusing on key terms. Abbreviations are usually perfectly acceptable in running titles. Thus the running title of a paper entitled 'Separation and identification of growth hormone variants with high-performance liquid chromatography techniques' could be 'HPLC separation of GH variants'.

7

Research papers: abstract

Nearly all original research papers have an abstract – a brief summary of the paper. It is the basis on which readers decide for or against reading the whole paper.

▲ Polish the abstract until it is just right

The abstract is usually the first part of a paper that editors and reviewers read. It is also the first, and sometimes the only, part of your paper that will be read by other scientists and clinicians. If the abstract is not clear, concise and informative, readers may not feel inclined to look any further into your paper. Therefore it pays to spend some time getting the abstract right – a well-written abstract may help get your paper published.

▲ Write the abstract after you have completed the paper

Usually, it is only after you have completed the paper that you will have thought sufficiently deeply about your key findings and their interpretation; so you will probably find it easiest to write the abstract last.

▲ If you do write the abstract first, revise it later

Some people find that writing a draft abstract before they sit down to write their paper helps them to plan the paper more effectively. Or you may already have written an abstract for a poster or presentation, and later write up the same data into a full paper. In that case, do not forget to revise the original draft abstract before you submit the paper – you will almost certainly want to make some changes.

▲ Do not exceed the stipulated length

Most Instructions to Authors stipulate a maximum length for the abstract – usually about 150–200 words. Even if no length is stipulated, keep it short. Some on-line databases cut off ('truncate') the abstract at 250 words, so anything longer is wasted.

▲ Check to see whether the journal uses structured abstracts

Some journals, particularly those that follow the CONSORT guidelines, use a structured abstract format. Subheadings are laid down by the journal, and might include, for example:

- Objective
- Design
- Setting
- Patients
- Primary outcome measures
- Results
- Conclusions.

▲ Use the structured abstract format to help you plan any abstract

If you need help deciding what to put into your abstract, and in what order, you can use the structured abstract format to help you plan. Then, when you have done this, just take the headings out and you have a well-planned ordinary abstract. However, don't try submitting a structured abstract to a journal that does not use this format – the copy-editor will simply take the headings out anyway.

▲ Write your abstract as one paragraph, unless it is a structured abstract or the Instructions to Authors say otherwise

Even though it might be more logical to divide up your abstract into paragraphs, most journals require abstracts (other than structured abstracts) to be written as one paragraph.

▲ Think about what you, as a reader, would like to find in the abstract

What are the most important questions you would want the abstract to answer? As Maeve O'Connor says in *How to Copy-edit Scientific Papers*: 'An abstract should answer the questions why did you start, what did you do, what answer did you get, and what does it mean anyway?'

▲ Make sure the abstract is self-contained …

The abstract should stand alone, without reference to the main body of the paper – remember, it will be read in isolation when it appears in a database.

▲ … And faithfully reflects the content of the paper

Never give any information in the abstract that is not included in the body of the paper.

▲ Always state the objective of the study

You will often see abstracts that jump straight into the study design. However, it is essential that readers know the objective of the study. What question were you asking when you began? As explained in Chapter 10, the objective and the method used to achieve it can be included in the same sentence, e.g. 'A randomized, placebo-controlled, double-blind study was conducted to determine …'

▲ If you have space, give a sentence or two of background before the objective

If you can afford the space, just one or two sentences establishing the context of the study will be helpful to readers who are unfamiliar with the current state of knowledge. For example, you could put 'Previous studies have shown … However, it is not known whether …' That would be just two sentences to set the scene. You could then go on to state the objective of the study: 'We therefore carried out a randomized, placebo-controlled, double-blind study to determine …' But do not waste space telling readers things they would almost certainly know, like 'Coronary heart disease is one of the commonest causes of death in the industrialized countries'.

▲ Give relevant details about the substances, tissues, species, subjects or patients included

To make an evaluation of the paper, readers need to know about the substances, tissues, species, subjects or patients used. They also need to know about their condition and, where appropriate, the sample size (e.g. '21 anaesthetized rats' or '205 diabetic men aged 16–65 years').

▲ Unless it is a 'methods' paper, keep the methods in the abstract brief

Unless the whole point of the paper is to describe a new method, detail should be kept to the minimum necessary to understand the results. But make sure you give the key information, without which the results would be meaningless (e.g. doses of drugs, duration of the study).

▲ The results of the study should comprise the bulk of the abstract

Readers are most interested in what you found in answer to the question you asked. So, in most abstracts, the results should take up most of the space. Think about which are the most important results and put them first. Pick out the most important pieces of data and use them, but beware of overwhelming the reader with endless strings of numbers.

▲ If you give percentages, make sure you also give the sample size

Readers need not just percentages but the sample size in order to make an informed judgement of the validity of the data. If the sample size does not vary, you need give it only once. If the sample size varies within the study, make this clear when you give the relevant data.

▲ If you give *p* values, make sure you give the actual data as well

It is not enough just to say 'Significantly more patients recovered in the treatment group than in the placebo group ($p < 0.05$)'. You need to give the actual data as well: 'Significantly more patients recovered in the treatment group than in the placebo group (86% vs 56%, $p < 0.05$).

▲ At the end of the abstract, briefly state the main conclusion

It helps the readers to know the 'bottom line', if there is one, e.g. 'This study shows that grottomycin is more effective than scabicillin in sinusitis in adults. It therefore offers a valuable new option in the management of this common condition'.

▲ State any *important* implications (optional)

If your findings are genuinely likely to change clinical practice, or change the whole way scientists look at the topic, there is no reason why you should not say so in the abstract. Otherwise, there is no need to say anything.

▲ Avoid non-standard abbreviations

All journals will allow you to use the standard abbreviations for SI units without spelling them out the first time they are used (e.g. g, L, cm). Most journals also have a standard list of other abbreviations which can be used without being spelled out (e.g. DNA, t.i.d.). Otherwise, only abbreviate a long term:

- if it is a widely recognised abbreviation
- if it is used repeatedly within the abstract.

For example, it is appropriate to abbreviate 'positron emission tomography' to 'PET' if it is used repeatedly in the abstract. This abbreviation is well known and saves a useful amount of space if it is used repeatedly. However, most journals would prefer you to spell out 'cefotaxime' rather than to abbreviate it to 'CTX', which is non-standard and saves very little space. If you use non-SI abbreviations, always spell them out the first time you use them, e.g. 'positron emission tomography (PET)'.

▲ Do not cite references in the abstract

Most journals have an absolute rule against citing references in the abstract. Very occasionally, you might be able to persuade them to make an exception, if citing a reference really does make life easier for the readers. For example, if the publication is a re-analysis of data from an earlier study, or a modification of a previously reported method, a reference would be useful. Note that the no references rule does not always apply to conference abstracts (see Chapter 8).

▲ Edit your abstract to eliminate wordiness

The first draft of your abstract is likely to be too long. Do not worry – thoroughly editing it according to the principle of clear, concise writing outlined in Chapters 24–26 will help you to reduce the number of words without losing any of the meaning.

- Use short sentences.
- Use short, simple words.
- Be very specific in your choice of words.
- Edit out all 'waste' words.
- Use the active voice wherever appropriate.
- Do not be afraid to use 'we'.

▲ Apply this reviewer's checklist to your abstract

Does the abstract:

- ❏ briefly establish the context, if space allows?
- ❏ state the main question you set out to answer?
- ❏ state the population or material studied?
- ❏ state the experimental approach or protocol used?
- ❏ state the most important results in logical order?
- ❏ state the main conclusion (the answer to the question)?
- ❏ give adequate data to support the conclusion?
- ❏ state any important implications (optional)?
- ❏ give a good overall impression – is the study well-conducted, interesting, worthwhile?

8

Conference abstracts

Most researchers will want to submit abstracts to scientific conferences to gain acceptance for an oral or poster presentation. These abstracts will be published in the form of an abstract book, which may itself be a part of a journal (and as such citeable as a reference).

Nearly all the rules given for writing abstracts as part of an original research paper apply to writing abstracts to appear in conference abstract books. However, there are some special points to note, as follows.

▲ A well-written abstract may help get your contribution accepted …

The content of the abstract will determine whether or not your contribution is accepted by the organizing committee. Some conferences have a policy of accepting nearly all abstracts submitted for publication in the abstract book, but also use abstracts to decide which contributions should be presented as posters or orally. The better the abstract, the better your chances of being asked to give a presentation. Selection committees look for good science – but if the abstract is confusingly written or incomplete, the standard of the research may be underestimated. A well-written abstract allows the scientific quality of a study to be assessed objectively.

▲ … And stimulate interest in your presentation or poster

During the conference itself, a clearly written abstract also encourages people to come to your talk or look at your poster.

▲ Get a copy of the instructions for submission of abstracts, and follow them carefully

Failure to follow the rules could result in your abstract being immediately returned to you for amendment, wasting the organizer's time and your own. Your abstract could even be rejected. Nowadays, abstracts are usually submitted via an electronic form on the organizer's website. This ensures that all abstracts can be published in a standard format.

▲ Edit your abstract thoroughly to make it fit

Ruthless editing for 'waste' words is often all you need to make a too-long abstract fit the space available.

▲ Consider using a graph or table if allowed

Journal abstracts never contain graphs or tables, mainly because these features cannot be included in on-line databases. However, some conference organizers are happy for you to include a graph or table in your conference abstract. This can be a nice way of displaying your data. The organizers will specify exactly how to insert graphs or tables in your abstract.

▲ You can use references in conference abstracts, if you really want to

In contrast to journal abstracts, there is no reason why you should not include one or two key references in a conference abstract, if you feel it is a worthwhile use of your limited space.

▲ Do not overdo the use of abbreviations

You have more leeway to use abbreviations in conference abstracts than in journal abstracts. Common abbreviations can be used without spelling them out on first use, unless the organizers say otherwise. But if you 'invent' an abbreviation to save space, spell it out on first use. However, spare a thought for your poor readers and do not over-use abbreviations. Abbreviations coined for the purpose of the abstract should be intuitively recognizable and not open to confusion with standard abbreviations. (Don't *you* hate the kind of conference abstract that says 'PDQ was used to compare the OP of ABC and XYZ at D3 in HB'?)

▲ Without results, your conference abstract may not be accepted …

It used to be common to see conference abstracts in the 'indicative' format. This format tells you what question the study was designed to answer, and something about the methods, but no results. You will probably have seen abstracts that begin 'Results will be presented for …' This gambit can be very useful for studies that are incomplete at the time of submission of the abstract. However, many organizing committees now refuse to accept such abstracts. They want to guard against the possibility that no results will be available for the meeting, and the abstract will have to be withdrawn. If you want to use an indicative abstract, it is advisable to check the organizing committee's policy.

▲ … But you can give interim results if necessary

It is, however, usually acceptable to give interim results – for example, for a small number of patients, or for just some of the variables you measured. If the organizers can be convinced that you will be in a position to present the full results at the meeting, they will be satisfied.

9

Research papers: introduction

The introduction describes why the research was done, and provides a context for the later discussion of the results. It allows readers to understand the background to the study, without having to consult the literature themselves.

▲ Remember that the introduction 'sells' the study

After reading the introduction, your readers should be convinced that your research is the next logical scientific step, and be keen to read on. As always, do not forget that readers include editors and reviewers as well as the wider scientific community. A well-written introduction can help to get your paper published by giving a good first impression, establishing your scientific credibility.

▲ Do not get stuck on the introduction

It is common for novice paper-writers to waste a lot of their time trying to get the introduction right before moving on to the rest of the paper. Ever spent hours trying to think of the first sentence? Many experienced authors write the introduction after the other main sections for two reasons:

1 it is easier to be clear-minded about why the study was necessary after you have put your own results in context with previous work in the discussion
2 writing the introduction last means that you are less likely to make it too long. No one wants to work hard writing text and then have to cut it.

▲ Limit the length of the introduction

Editors often complain that introductions are too long. You only need provide enough information to help readers understand the reasons for the study. The introduction is not a wide-ranging review of your field of research. Look at your chosen journal to check the typical length of introduction relative to the rest of the paper. Often, it will be no more than one-eighth or one-tenth of the total length. Half a printed page or 400–500 words is also a good guide.

▲ Do not overinflate the introduction at the expense of the discussion

Do not forget that in the discussion you will have the opportunity to compare and contrast the findings of your study with those of other researchers . If you go into too much detail about other researchers' findings in the introduction, you will end up repeating yourself in the discussion.

▲ Select references carefully

Cite only those references that are truly relevant. This is not your PhD thesis – you do not need to prove how well read you are.

▲ Use the present tense for generalizations

Use the present tense for generalizations, and a past/present combination for specific findings that are now established fact. For example:

- generalization: 'Repetitive strain injury (RSI) **is** [present tense] one of the commonest complications of writing a thesis.[1]'
- specific finding: 'The Postgraduate Writers' Trial **has shown** [past tense] that use of a wrist rest **reduces** [present tense] the risk of RSI.[2]'

In both of these examples, the use of the present tense is a convention to indicate established fact. In effect, it means that we are convinced that the findings of the Postgraduate Writers' Trial are valid.

▲ Use the past tense for specific findings with which you are about to take issue

It is acceptable to use the past tense for specific findings of others that are not considered established fact, e.g. 'Smith and Brown **reported** [past tense] that the moon was made of green cheese.[3] However, other studies have not confirmed this finding.[4-5]'

▲ Begin the introduction with what is known

Start off by briefly summarizing relevant current knowledge of the topic, supporting your statements with references as necessary.

▲ Move on to what is not known (or a problem with the known)

Having summarized the established facts, move on to areas where there is less or no knowledge, or where the evidence is conflicting.

▲ End the introduction by stating the question

Every study sets out to answer a specific question, which is stated explicitly in the introduction. Make sure the question follows logically from the preceding sentences. State the question carefully because you will be coming back to it later when you show how your results answer the question.

▲ State the question in a new paragraph

Stating the question in a new paragraph – the last paragraph of the introduction – attracts attention. Readers naturally look to the last paragraph of the introduction to find the question.

▲ Use 'signalling' words and phrases to highlight the question

Examples include:

• 'However, it is not known whether ...'

- 'To answer this question we …'
- 'To clarify the role of A in B, we …'
- 'To determine whether …'
- To compare the efficacy of X and Y in Z, we …'

Note the use of active verbs such as *clarify, determine, compare, establish, verify, find out* in the statement of the question.

▲ Very briefly, state how you set out to answer the question

After stating the question, give very brief details of how you set out to answer it – this will help emphasize the rationale for the study, and set the scene for the methods section to follow. Mention the experimental method and the species, material or patient group as appropriate.

▲ The question and what was done to answer it can often be combined

Often, you can go straight on from the question to the experimental method, e.g. 'To compare the efficacy of grottomycin with scabicillin in sinusitis, we conducted a multicentre, double-blind randomized trial in adults'. But beware of writing excessively long sentences.

▲ Always state the question in the present tense and what was done to answer it in the past tense

'To determine whether X **is** effective in Y, we **conducted** a double-blind, placebo-controlled study in …'

▲ Clearly separate minor questions from the main question

There may be subsidiary questions that you set out to answer. If so, state these in one or more separate sentences, e.g. 'We also investigated the effects of C on D'.

▲ The introduction tells a story – make sure it has a logical flow

The introduction needs to provide a convincing justification for your reasearch. Make sure your readers understand the connections between one part of the story and another. Underline the logic with signalling words and phrases such as:

'**Thus**, it appears that ...'; '**It was previously believed that ...**'; '**However**, recent studies have shown ...'

▲ Do not be afraid to say what is new and important about the study

Your introduction helps to 'sell' the paper to readers and reviewers; so do not be afraid to state what is new or important about it. There is no need to be boastful – just state the facts, e.g. 'Placebo-controlled pilot studies have shown grottomycin to be clinically and microbiologically effective in acute sinusitis in adults, but so far no comparisons with other agents have been reported. We therefore conducted a multicentre, double-blind randomized trial to compare the efficacy of grottomycin with that of the standard treatment, scabicillin'.

▲ Apply this reviewer's checklist to your introduction

Does the introduction:

❏ identify a gap in scientific knowledge?
❏ show why the study was necessary?
❏ state the question clearly?
❏ briefly summarize the approach?
❏ show what is new and important about the study?
❏ 'sell' the study?

10

Research papers: methods

This section of a research paper may be entitled just *Methods*, or *Materials and methods* or *Patients and methods*, depending on the journal. Its function is to allow interested readers to judge the validity of your results in the context of the methods used. It is equivalent to a 'recipe' for the investigation.

▲ Remember the 'acid test' – repeatability

The classical test of a methods section is that it should be sufficiently detailed to allow competent investigators to repeat the study, should they wish to do so. This means that the methods should be comprehensive, while avoiding fussy, irrelevant detail.

▲ Write the methods section first

Usually, the methods section is the easiest to write – you may even have some of it ready-written in the form of a protocol. Writing the easiest part of the paper first will begin to focus your mind on the results linked to the methods. It will also give you confidence, as you will have got a substantial part of the paper finished, usually quite quickly and easily.

▲ Make the methods as long as they need to be – but no longer

To meet the criterion of repeatability, the methods section often has to be quite long. This is not necessarily a problem – it is common for the methods to take up a third or more of the paper. However, if you find they are more than half the length of the paper, you should consider whether all the detail is strictly necessary. You might well decide that it *is* justified – it all depends on the type of study. Note that some journals allow you to include additional detail on methods in supplementary information available online.

▲ Just summarize the methods if they have been described in another paper

Occasionally, the methods of your study will have already been described in detail in another publication. For example, some large, multicentre clinical studies publish their methods in a separate paper at the outset of the study. Subsequent papers originating from such studies should just give a brief summary of the methods – enough to enable readers to understand the content of the paper – and a reference.

▲ Describe only methods for which you later give a result

List only those methods for which you will later give a result. In this respect, the methods of a research paper differs from that of a thesis or clinical trial report, in which everything you either did or planned to do may be described for completeness – even if no result was obtained. In a paper, you can leave out a method if it yielded no result for some technical reason. You cannot of course leave out a method simply because the result did not fit in with your hypothesis!

▲ Write the methods in a logical order

The convention usually used is:

1 materials, animals, subjects or patients (often nowadays called 'participants')
2 study design (including randomization)
3 observational and experimental methods
4 statistical methods used to evaluate the significance of the results.

If you think about it, this is more or less the same sequence in which research is carried out – you cannot start until you have decided which animals, subjects or patients to work on, you cannot undertake any observations or measurements until you have designed the study and so on.

▲ Clinical trials also follow the standard order

Clinical trial reports also follow a standard order, which is typically broken down into:

1 participant recruitment
2 inclusion/exclusion criteria
3 method of randomization
4 primary outcomes
5 secondary outcomes
6 adverse events monitoring
7 statistical methods

Consult the CONSORT statement for further information (www.consort-statement.org).

▲ Prefer logical order to strict chronological order

Although you write the methods in roughly the same order as you did the research, there is no need to follow a strict chronological order. This is unnecessary and may be confusing. Often, we do things in a certain order simply for convenience. For example, you may only have been able to gain access to equipment at certain times. The methods section should flow logically, rather than being simply a diary of what you did.

▲ Use subheadings if needed

Long methods sections benefit from the use of subheadings to help readers find their way around. Most journals provide for the use of subheadings of your own choice, such as *Study design, Patient selection, Treatments, Outcome measures, Statistical methods* and so on.

▲ Use tables or flow charts if required

There is no reason why tables and flow charts should be confined to the results section – most journals will let you use them in the methods if you need to. For example, a flow chart may be useful in describing a complex study design, or a table in listing strains of micro-organisms and their origin. Remember, however, the rules for using tables and illustrations given in Chapters 12 and 13. Journals will not accept them if they feel the information could have been presented just as well in the text.

▲ Answer the questions readers (and reviewers) will want to ask

Imagine the questions that would be going through an informed colleague's mind about 'How many?', 'How much?' and 'How long?', and aim to provide precise answers.

▲ Write the methods in the past tense

As you are describing what you did, rather than stating established fact, it is correct to use the past tense throughout the methods.

▲ 'We' is usually acceptable and adds variety

Most journals are happy for you to use 'we' (meaning the researchers) in an active construction, e.g. 'We measured lower leg growth using a knemometer' as an alternative to the traditional passive construction 'Lower leg growth was measured using a knemometer'. This can add variety to the methods section. Beware, however, of writing something that sounds like a child's description of a day at the seaside: 'We did this. We did that. We did something else.'

▲ Do not describe established techniques in detail

Novel techniques, or variants on old ones, should be described in detail. However, if you followed an established method, you only need to describe it briefly. Use your judgement regarding whether a reference is necessary – do readers *need* a reference to enable them to look up and follow the technique? There is no need to discuss or provide references for statistical techniques unless they are unusual.

▲ In clinical trials, distinguish between primary and secondary outcome measures

It is usual to have one primary measure of efficacy and perhaps a number of secondary ones. For example, in a trial of corticosteroids in asthma, the primary outcome measure might be 'percentage change in morning peak expiratory flow rate (PEFR) compared with baseline'. Secondary outcome measures might include 'use of bronchodilators' and 'patient's subjective rating of efficacy of treatment'. Primary outcome measures (sometimes called primary efficacy variables) are always described before secondary measures.

▲ In studies on humans, remember to state compliance with ethical regulations

This statement usually goes at the end of the section describing the participant recruitment and selection. A typical statement would be: 'The trial protocol was approved by the Ethical Committee of the University Hospital of Wherever, and the trial was conducted in accordance with the Declaration of Helsinki. All patients gave informed consent.'

▲ Include relevant statistical information

Make sure you include all the relevant statistical information:

- *statistical tests.* You need not give references for common tests, but you should give references for any unusual techniques
- *method of randomization.* This often used to be omitted, but many journals now require it. You can be very brief, e.g. 'Patients were allocated to treatment and placebo groups using a blinded randomization list'
- *power of the study.* Where appropriate, describe any power calculations you carried out to determine appropriate sample sizes for your study
- p *value taken to indicate statistical significance.* Although it is often assumed that a *p* value of 0.05 or less indicates statistical significance, statisticians prefer you to make this absolutely clear.

▲ In clinical trials, patient baseline data go in the results, not the methods

One common mistake of which editors complain is the inclusion of patient baseline data (sometimes called demographic data) in the methods section. Examples of such data include age, weight, sex and so on. Usually a comparison is made to find out if there were any significant differences in baseline characteristics between groups at the start of the study. All these observations, measurements and calculations are made on patients who you have already decided to include in the study and are therefore results and not methods.

▲ Use 'measured', 'calculated' and 'estimated' precisely

Be precise about what you actually did to obtain the numbers given in the results. You can use 'determined' to cover the mixed process of measuring and calculating. Avoid the use of vague terms like 'evaluated' when there is a more precise alternative.

▲ Make relationships between parts of the sample clear

If you only performed certain measurements or procedures on part of the sample, make this clear, e.g. 'PET scanning was performed on four of the 11 subjects in the drug treatment group and five of the 13 subjects in the placebo group'.

▲ Be concise

The methods section may be quite long, but that does not mean that you can afford to waste space. Avoid 'waste' words, repetition and fussy detail that is not relevant to the repeatability of the study.

▲ Apply this reviewer's checklist to your methods

Do the methods:

❑ clearly describe how the question was approached?
❑ give necessary detail about any animals used, e.g. species, housing, age, weight?
❑ state the method of randomization (often neglected)?
❑ state planned group sizes?
❑ give inclusion and exclusion criteria for participants?
❑ give necessary details of materials?
❑ state precise drug dose regimens?
❑ use up-to-date and appropriate techniques?
❑ use an appropriate means of statistical analysis (chosen *a priori*)?
❑ give an estimate of the power of the study?
❑ state the p value used to disprove the null hypothesis?
❑ make clear which question is addressed by which method?
❑ provide sufficient information to allow repetition by another scientist?

11
Research papers: results

The function of the results section is to present the data obtained during the study. The results section is the 'core' of the paper, even though it can be quite short. It is often the first place that readers familiar with the topic will look (after the title and abstract). Readers expect the results to provide them with enough data to draw their own conclusions about the answer to the question posed in the introduction.

▲ Match the results to the methods

For every result that you describe, there should be a method and vice versa. Check each section and make sure that there are no 'unmatched' results or methods. The results follow the same order as the methods – if you have ordered your methods logically, the results will also be in logical order.

▲ The results usually follow a standard order

The typical order of the results, which mirrors the standard order of the methods, is:

1 baseline data
2 effectiveness of randomization (where relevant)
3 observational and experimental data from most important to least important.

An expanded version of this standard order is given for the results of clinical trials (see below).

▲ There is a standard way of presenting the results of clinical trials

In clinical trials, the standard order of the results is usually as follows:

1 baseline data (sometimes called demographic data)
2 effectiveness of randomization
3 patients included in the analysis (intention to treat/fully evaluable patients)
4 primary outcome measures
5 secondary outcome measures
6 adverse events
7 deaths.

There are exceptions, of course – for example, a trial might compare two agents of equal efficacy in terms of their side-effects, in which case 'adverse events' would be the primary outcome measure.

▲ Use subheadings in long results sections

As in the methods section, subheadings can help readers to find their way around a long results section. You might like to use separate subheadings to distinguish between outcome measure, e.g. 'Five-year survival', 'Costs of treatment'. Smaller subheadings can be used where necessary for further subdivision, e.g. 'Control group', 'Treatment group' or 'Men, Women'.

▲ Match results subheadings to methods subheadings

If you used subheadings in your methods section, you can go on to use the same subheadings (where relevant) in the results.

▲ Focus on results that help to answer the question

Your results should be mainly composed of data that help to answer the question posed in the introduction. This means that you *must* report your predetermined primary and secondary outcome measures.

▲ You do not have to include every piece of data you obtained

You do not have to report all the data collected, only that which is relevant and representative. The mere fact that you measured something does not force you to include it in your results. Data that do not help to answer the question can be excluded, or summarized in a sentence or two. For example, most drug trials collect extensive biochemical and haematological data. If nothing untoward is observed, it is usually enough to say 'No clinically relevant abnormalities were seen in routine biochemical and haematological testing'.

▲ Include results whether or not they support your hypothesis

Although it is permissible to select results in terms of leaving out irrelevant or incomplete data, it is certainly not permissible to leave out results simply because they do not give you the answer you want.

▲ Use tables and figures wherever appropriate, especially for important results

Many readers look at the tables and figures first to try and get the gist of the results; so, if data can be presented more effectively in tables or figures, do so. There are four good reasons for using a table or figure:

1 it is the only reasonable way of presenting the data (e.g. you cannot describe a curve)
2 it is the easiest way to understand the data (e.g. change over time)
3 it is the most space-efficient way of presenting the data (e.g. large tables would require a great deal of text space to describe their content)
4 it highlights the most important findings (e.g. a bar chart to demonstrate dramatic differences between study groups). Many editors do not regard 'emphasis' as sufficient reason to use a figure or table.

▲ Do not submit more tables and graphs than the journal is likely to accept

Many journals have a rule that you cannot use tables or graphs to represent data that could have been given more concisely in the text. As E J Huth says in *How to Write and Publish Papers in the Medical Sciences*: 'Editors must hold down numbers of tables and illustrations because of their high cost and potential difficulties in layout.' So be prepared to select among the many tables and graphs that could be used to illustrate your results, and choose those that are essential. Look at the journal to see what ratio of figures and tables to text seems acceptable – some journals actually specify 'no more than X figures or tables' in the Instructions to Authors. Many journals now allow you to supply additional figures and tables as supplementary data available online.

▲ Do not repeat large amounts of data from tables and graphs in the text

Most journals' Instructions to Authors warn against repetition of data from tables and graphs in the text.

▲ Make general statements, then back them up with specific data

Do not be afraid to state the 'obvious'. This saves work for the reader, and helps them to distinguish the key points in your paper. For example, it is more helpful to say 'Mean time to recovery was significantly faster in the treatment group than in the placebo group (6.5 vs 14.1 days, $p < 0.05$)', rather than just 'Mean time to recovery was 6.5 days in the treatment group and 14.1 days in the placebo group'.

▲ If there were no significant differences, there is no need to give p values

It is usually enough to say 'There were no significant differences between the treatments for outcome measures A, B and C' rather than to give p values for each comparison. However, if you were including p values in a table, you would include them whether or not they showed significant differences.

▲ Emphasize important differences

You can report percentage change or percentage difference as well as (but not instead of) exact data.

▲ Give results for experimental groups before those for control groups

It is conventional to give results for experimental groups first, to make comparison easier for readers. Thus, you would put: 'The mean clinical cure rate at two weeks was 98% in the treatment group and 54% in the placebo group' and not 'The mean clinical cure rate at two weeks was 54% in the placebo group and 98% in the treatment group'.

▲ Remember to give confidence intervals/standard deviation and sample size

When comparing means, it is usual to give confidence intervals (CI)/standard deviation (SD) and sample size as well as *p* values. Check past copies of the journal for how confidence limits and standard deviations should be expressed. If in doubt, take advice from a statistician.

▲ If the sample size varies, give actual numbers after percentages

Even if readers could work out the sample size from information given elsewhere in the text, it is helpful for them to see it next to the data, e.g. 'Of the patients receiving scabicillin, 46% (17/37) reported one or more adverse events'.

▲ Always refer to figures and tables in the text

Make sure that every figure and table you include is mentioned in the text. The standard practice is to put figure and table citations in brackets at the end of the first sentence stating the relevant result, e.g. 'The mean clinical cure rate at two weeks was 98% in the treatment group and 54% in the placebo group (Figure 1)'. Do not put 'see Figure 1' or 'Figure 1, below' – if you do, the journal's copy-editor will edit out the excess words.

▲ It is acceptable to put data in brackets after stating the result they support

Giving a general statement of the result, followed by specific data in brackets, is an economical way of presenting results. For example, you could put: 'The incidence of diarrhoea was significantly lower in the grottomycin group than in the scabicillin group (14% vs 38%, $p = 0.021$).'

▲ Generally speaking, readers will assume 'significant' refers to statistics

Just say 'significant difference' or 'significantly different' to denote statistical significance; there is rarely any need to say 'statistically significant difference'. Generally speaking, editors do not like the use of the term 'clinically significant', as it has the potential to cause confusion. Prefer 'clinically relevant' or 'clinically important' instead.

▲ Avoid vague comparisons, or those that make value judgements

Be specific – what does 'increased markedly' really mean? It would be better to put 'increased by 100%', or 'doubled' or 'twice the effect'.

▲ Write all of the results in the past tense

The results describe what was found in one particular study rather than established fact, and should all be in the past tense.

▲ Do not be tempted to discuss the results unless the journal combines Results with Discussion

However tempting it may be to give each result and then to discuss what it means, this is not the norm in biomedical papers. Some basic science journals do have combined Results and Discussion sections. Normally, however, a strict distinction should be drawn between saying what you found and discussing what it means. You should not attempt to draw conclusions, nor to relate your findings to the work of others.

▲ Do not include references in the results section

Since the results must only report what you found, it is not appropriate to refer to the work of others.

▲ Apply this reviewer's checklist to your results

Do the results:

❏ establish the comparability of groups?
❏ give both the size and significance of differences?
❏ give means to no more than one additional decimal point than that of original measurement?
❏ give means with sample size, range, SD and/or CI where appropriate?
❏ give analyses of variance with degrees of freedom and F values where appropriate?
❏ include appropriate figures and tables?
❏ not repeat data given in figures and tables in text (except for key data)?
❏ present but not discuss data?
❏ avoid misleading statements (e.g. 'X was larger than Y but the difference failed to achieve statistical significance')?

12

Research papers: figures

The term 'figures', as used by biomedical journals, may include:

- graphs (e.g. line graphs, scattergrams)
- charts (e.g. vertical or horizontal bar graphs, pie charts)
- photographs (black and white or colour)
- micrographs/electron micrographs
- electrophoretograms (photographs of gels)
- polygraph recordings (e.g. ECG, EEG)
- line drawings (e.g. flow charts, surgical procedures).

Photographs have their own separate list of tips (see Chapter 14).

▲ Remember that figures are often the first thing that readers look at

Readers (including reviewers) often look at figures first to make a preliminary assessment of the results, so they have to make a good first impression.

▲ Avoid unnecessary figures

Do not use a figure if the data could be represented by a simple sentence or two. For example, a bar chart with only two bars may be acceptable as a slide, but if you included the same chart in a paper, many journals would reject it on the grounds of space. They would argue that the same data could have been more concisely represented in the text.

▲ Be prepared to be selective

Even if you have half-a-dozen relevant, interesting figures, the journal may not be prepared to publish them all. Some journals set limits on the number of figures they will accept, others leave it to your discretion. As a rough guide, one figure or table per 1000 words of text will probably be accepted without quibbling. As mentioned in Chapter 11, you may be able to include extra figures in the online version of your paper.

▲ Do not expect the journal to publish the same data in both figure and table form ...

Submit your data in whichever form is most appropriate.

▲ ... But be prepared to submit backup data for figures

Some journals now request that figures be backed up with tables showing the raw data used to construct them. This is to save reviewers the trouble of trying to establish values for data points that are just represented as spots on a graph. Just because you have to supply the raw data, however, does not mean that it will be published. Look at the Instructions to Authors to see whether this requirement applies.

▲ Provide figures in the format requested by the journal

Check the Instructions to Authors for acceptable formats for figures. Most request electronic files in a specified format that can be incorporated directly into the journal without redrawing. A few top journals redraw the figures to their house style.

▲ Do not try to fit too much information onto one graph

Think about how much information the readers will be able to take in. For example, line graphs with more than four lines are likely to be too difficult to read, especially if the lines overlap.

▲ Make sure the lettering is large enough

Think about how much your figure will have to be reduced to fit into a single column. Then work out what the reduced height of the letters will be. Usually, the reduced size of a lower-case letter without ascenders or descenders should be no less than 2 mm, or it will be too difficult to read.

▲ Make sure that symbols will still be distinguishable after reproduction

Remember that it may be difficult to tell the difference between microscopically small circles, squares or triangles. Make sure that they will be at least 2 mm high after reduction. The standard symbols used by most journals are circles (●/○), usually followed by triangles and squares.

▲ Emphasize the data, not the axes

The thickest lines should be used for curves or plots, thinner lines for axes and error bars. Most scientific graphics programs will take care of this for you.

▲ Do not extend the axes too far

The X and Y axes should extend only to the next 'tick mark' on the axis after the maximum values for the data. Again, your graphics programme will probably take care of this for you.

▲ Indicate significant differences between points with asterisks

It is standard practice to draw attention to significant differences on graphs with asterisks, the meanings of which are defined in footnotes. A standard series is $*p < 0.05$; $**p < 0.01$; $***p < 0.001$, but check with the journal.

▲ Check where keys to symbols should be placed

The Instructions to Authors usually include advice on where to put the keys to symbols used on your graphs. Usually, the key is given on the graph itself, but a very few journals put them in the figure title (also known as the figure legend).

▲ Define abbreviations if used

Generally, figure legends should be understandable without reference to the text. Usually, abbreviations used in figures should be defined below the figure title even if you have already defined them in the text, but check with the Instructions to Authors. If you use the same abbreviations in several figures, it is common practice to define them in the first one and then cross refer, e.g. 'For abbreviations, see Figure 1', or 'Abbreviations as in Figure 1'.

▲ Supply figure titles on a separate file

Figure titles must be supplied in a separate file to the figure itself as they will go through separate production processes. Figure titles follow a similar format to that for tables (see Chapter 13).

▲ If you use someone else's figure, it is your responsibility to get written permission

If you want to reproduce a figure first given by another author in an original publication, you will have to get permission in writing. It is your responsibility to do this, not the publisher's. You should write to the managing editor of the journal in which the figure first appeared, asking permission to reproduce it. Say where you plan to reuse it. The journal will usually respond giving you permission, and stating a set form of words to be used for acknowledgement, e.g. 'Reproduced with permission from …' Often, you will be asked to write to the original author as well. A few journals may ask for payment for reproduction of figures, and some impose rules on whether they can be redrawn or adapted in any way.

▲ Make sure your figure is referred to in the text

Check that for every figure, there is a reference in the text ('Figure 1' or 'Fig. 1'), and vice versa. You should also indicate approximately where the figure should appear, by a note in the text (clearly distinguished from the text to be printed).

▲ Apply this reviewer's checklist to your figures

Do the figures:

❏ show data in the most appropriate and efficient way?
❏ show important data?
❏ show what the text says they show?
❏ have appropriate explanatory titles?
❏ explain any abbreviations, symbols and shading used?
❏ avoid distracting extraneous detail?
❏ include error bars where appropriate?

13

Research papers: tables

Use tables to demonstrate the relationships between numerical and/or descriptive data. A good table can compress a lot of information into a small space, yet make the meaning crystal clear.

▲ Avoid unnecessary tables

Do not use a table if the data could be presented better as a graph, or if they could be given more concisely in the text – if you use unnecessary tables, the journal may well edit them out.

▲ Follow the Instructions to Authors carefully

Most journals give detailed instructions on how tables are to be set out.

▲ Type each table and its title on a separate page

To make life easier for the journal's production department, each table should appear on a separate page. These pages go either at the end of the manuscript, or in a separate file, according to journal requirements. The title should be typed above the table. Even though you may think it more logical to insert tables in the text – do not – most journals will send your paper straight back to you.

▲ Use the tables function on your word processor, if the journal allows

The tables function in word-processing software such as Word makes the creation of tables a painless process. However, check the Instructions to Authors – a few specify particular formatting rules to ensure compatability with their own software.

▲ Use horizontal lines to define key areas of the table

Most journals require you to use horizontal lines to separate the column headings from the body of the table, and to delineate the top and bottom of the table. It is also permissible to use horizontal lines to separate column headings from subheadings. Within the body of the table, most journals use spaces rather than lines to mark groups of row headings.

▲ Do not use vertical lines in tables in papers

Most journals do not permit you to use vertical lines within tables, however useful you think they may be. This is really a hangover from older systems of typesetting that meant that setting of vertical lines was difficult and time-consuming. Although setting vertical lines is easier nowadays, you should always follow the journal's instructions.

▲ Do not try to pack too much data into one table

You do not have to include every variable that you measured. Select those that readers need to know in order to evaluate the answer to the question. Each table should represent just one key idea or message.

▲ Arrange tables so that important comparisons are made from left to right

Most readers are accustomed to reading tables from left to right, not top to bottom. This makes the table easier to read and understand (see the example below).

This way ...

	Grottomycin 50 mg b.d. (n = 108)	Scabicillin 5 g t.i.d. (n = 111)	p
Clinical cure (%)	87.9	60.3	$p < 0.05$
Microbiological cure (%)	79.6	59.4	$p < 0.05$

... rather than this way

	Clinical cure (%)	Microbiological cure (%)
Grottomycin 50 mg b.d. (n = 108)	87.9	79.6
Scabicillin 5 g t.i.d. (n = 111)	60.3	59.4
p	<0.05	<0.05

▲ Align the column and row headings according to the journal's requirements

Usually, the row headings should be aligned flush left, and the column headings centred. The contents of the columns are usually centred over the decimal point.

▲ Make the table self-contained

Readers will often look at the tables first to get the key points of the results without having to plough through lots of text. So make sure that the table and its title contain the key information the reader needs.

▲ Keep column headings short

A maximum of two lines is a good general rule. If necessary, use abbreviations and define them in footnotes (but see below).

▲ Make sure you include units of measure, where appropriate

Column and row headings should include units of measure (SI), usually in brackets (check with the journal for the correct style).

▲ Use non-SI abbreviations only if necessary, and define them in a footnote

Readers do not want to search through your paper looking for the meaning of abbreviations. So, even if you have abbreviated a term elsewhere in the paper, try to spell it out where it is used in the column or row headings, unless it is very long. If you have to use non-SI abbreviations, define them in a footnote to the table.

▲ Do not let footnotes take over your table

If your list of footnotes is taking over the table, think again. Readers do not want to have to fight their way through a mass of abbreviations to understand your table. Could you spell out at least some of the shorter terms instead of abbreviating them?

▲ Define abbreviations in the first table, then cross-refer (but check journal style)

If you use the same abbreviations in several tables, it is common practice to define them in the first one and then cross-refer, e.g. 'For abbreviations, see Table 1', or 'Abbreviations as in Table 1'.

▲ Indent row subheadings

Row subheadings should be indented, as in the next tip.

▲ Give row headings and subheadings a logical order

Rather than just put your row headings down in the order you first thought of, think about what order will make the data easiest to interpret. If you have a lot of row headings, grouping them will make the data easier to understand. For example:

> *Drug costs*
> > *Anti-emetics*
> > *Sedatives*
>
> *Administration costs*
> > *Disposables*
> > *Physician time*
> > *Nursing time*

▲ Use only meaningful decimal places

Ask yourself how accurately you measured each variable. Means should be given to, at most, one decimal place more than in the original measurements.

▲ Be consistent with decimal places

Use the same number of decimal places in all values for one variable. Use the same number of decimal places in standard deviations, standard errors or confidence intervals as in the mean.

▲ Be careful about the use of percentages

The use of percentages is particularly helpful when sample size varies between groups. However, some journals only allow percentages for sample sizes of 50 or more. Others require that the sample should be as large as 100. Check with the Instructions to Authors for guidance.

▲ You can give both numbers and percentages in the same column

For the reader's convenience, it is often appropriate to include both numbers and percentages in the same column, like this.

> Clinical cure at 4 wk
> n (%)
> _____
> 47/58 (81)

▲ Do not leave cells blank

Leaving cells blank leaves the reader guessing – was the value zero, or was it just not successfully measured? Follow the journal's style for missing data. A typical style is:

0.0	the value was zero
–	the value was not measured or is not given for some other reason.

Other abbreviations you may see are:

ND	the value was not determined
NA	the value is not available

Any abbreviations or symbols used should be defined in footnotes.

▲ You can indicate statistical significance with p values or footnote indicators

You may want to give p values in a separate column (see above). Alternatively, you can save space if you use asterisks, defined in footnotes. A standard series is $*p < 0.05$; $**p < 0.01$; $***p < 0.001$, but check with the journal.

▲ Use the journal's standard hierarchy of footnote indicators

As mentioned above, asterisks are usually used to denote statistical significance. Other footnote indicators are sometimes also used. These may be:

Symbols	e.g. †, ‡, §, ll, ¶, #, **, ††
Letters	[a], [b], [c]
Numbers	[1], [2], [3] (normally only used where the journal style does not include numbered references).

▲ Check and recheck your numbers

Make sure columns that are supposed to add up to 100% do so. Make sure that all parts of the sample are accounted for.

▲ Make sure all data given in tables coincide with values given in the text

It is annoying to readers to find a value of 27% given in a table and 26% given in the text, yet it is all too easy to make amendments to the tables without amending the text and vice versa. Check which numbers are correct and try to be absolutely consistent.

▲ Give the table a descriptive title

The reader should be able to understand the table without searching for the relevant section of text. The table title should typically include:

- independent variable(s)
- dependent variable(s)
- species or patients studied

Thus a typical table title might be 'Table 2. Clinical and microbiological efficacy of grottomycin and scabicillin in adults with sinusitis'.

Tables containing other types of data will not have all these components in the title, but should follow a similar pattern, e.g. 'Table 1. Baseline characteristics of patients at randomization'.

▲ Keep the table title short – usually

Most journals prefer titles of one to three lines. However, a few put more emphasis on the 'tables must be self-contained' principle than on brevity – in *Nature*, for example, the table titles contain so much information they may take up more space than the table itself. Follow the usual style of the journal, but be as concise as you can – do not waste words, even in a long table title.

▲ Think about how many columns the table will occupy

Look at the journal, and think about whether your table will occupy just one text column, or whether it will take the full width of the page. This may influence the number of columns you decide to include in the table. If you have just a little too much data for one column, it can look rather thinly spread over two.

▲ Use 'sideways' tables only if they are very important

You will sometimes see tables taking up a whole page on their own, laid out at right angles to the rest of the text. Use this format only if the table is very important, and you are sure the journal will allow it. In review articles, for example, this may be the most efficient way of comparing a number of different studies. Some journals will insist that all tables have to be read from the top to bottom of the page in the normal way. If they think you have too much data in a large table, they may ask you to edit some out or subdivide the table.

▲ Make sure your table is referred to in the text

Check that for every table there is a reference in the text ('Table 1'), and vice versa. You should also indicate to the editor approximately where the table should appear, by a note in the margin.

▲ Apply this reviewer's checklist to your tables

Do the tables:

❑ match journal style?
❑ each deal with a specific question?
❑ have a clear and uncomplicated layout?
❑ show what the text says they show?
❑ include appropriate explanatory titles?
❑ give actual data as well as percentages?
❑ avoid using excessive numbers of decimal points?
❑ avoid irrelevant detail?
❑ include SD, CI and p values where appropriate?
❑ add up correctly (i.e. no missing or extra numbers)?
❑ explain abbreviations and symbols used?

14

Research papers: photographs

You may want to include photographs in a paper or article. For example, you may have clinical photographs showing the manifestations of a disease (perhaps before and after treatment). You may also want to publish radiographs or scans, photomicrographs or electronmicrographs.

▲ Preparing photographs correctly saves time and errors

Knowing how to prepare photographic images in a form acceptable to the journal will save unnecessary exchanges of letters between you and the managing editor, and thus avoid delays in publication. It will also help to ensure that photographs appear exactly as you intended.

▲ Supply photographs in the format requested by the journal

Nowadays photographs are usually supplied as electronic files. Follow the journal's instructions regarding the file format.

▲ Check whether the journal accepts colour photographs, and on what terms

Most journals accept black and white photographs, but some do not accept colour photographs at all. Others limit the number of colour photographs you can submit, while some expect you to pay a fee for each colour photograph (even though you do not pay a fee for publication of the paper itself). Paying for colour photographs is common, for example, in histology journals.

▲ Make sure photographs are good enough to be printed

A poor-resolution photograph will not look any better when printed in the journal than it does on your computer screen.

▲ Make sure photographs are clearly identified by figure number

Name your photographic files to avoid misunderstanding. This is especially important if several similar photographs are submitted.

▲ Crop photographs to eliminate unwanted parts

If you only want part of a photograph to be printed, crop it yourself before you submit the file.

▲ Mask patients' eyes where necessary

In most journals, it is standard practice to put a black bar across patients' eyes to avoid identification.

▲ Obtain a signed consent form from patients and pass it on to the journal

Most journals request that you obtain permission from patients to use their photographs, whether or not their faces appear, and whether or not their eyes will be masked. It is your responsibility to obtain this permission in writing from the patient (or, in the case of a child, their parent or legal guardian). Failure to do so could result in costly legal action at a later date. How would you like it if someone used your photograph without permission to illustrate a disease?

▲ Remember to remove patients' names from radiographs and scans

Cut off or mask patients' names when they appear on radiographs or scans.

▲ Remember to mark arrows and labels on the photograph

You should add arrows or labels such as A, B on the photograph. Don't expect the journal to do this for you.

▲ Type titles on a separate page

As with all figure titles, titles of photographs should be included with the figure legends, which are usually supplied in a separate file. The title always begins with a figure number, e.g. 'Figure 1. Cross-section of ...'

▲ Make sure your photograph is referred to in the text

Make sure that for every photograph there is a reference in the text ('Figure 1'), and vice versa. You should also indicate to the editor approximately where the photograph should appear, by a note in the text (clearly distinguished from the text to be printed).

15

Research papers: discussion and conclusions

The functions of the discussion section of an original research paper (sometimes divided into discussion and conclusions) are to:

- answer the question posed in the introduction
- explain how the results support the answer
- put the results into context.

▲ Write your discussion to anticipate the readers' and reviewers' questions

The discussion acts like a dialogue with interested readers, answering all the questions they are likely to ask. It is important to write the discussion carefully, because papers have been known to be rejected because of a poor discussion. As one reviewer said: 'If authors do not know what their own results mean, it is not my job to tell them.'

▲ Plan your discussion logically

The discussion needs to be well structured if it is to be convincing to readers and reviewers. You can use the planning techniques in Chapter 5 to construct a discussion that is logical and easy for the reader to follow. This will give the best possible support to your results.

▲ Begin by stating the answer to the question, i.e. the conclusion

You should begin the discussion by answering the question (i.e. stating the conclusion) in exactly the same way that you asked it. For example:

Introduction: 'We conducted a double-blind, placebo-controlled study to compare inhaled thingerol, 50 g b.d., with inhaled wotsiterol, 200 mg q.i.d., in the control of nocturnal symptoms in asthma.'
Discussion: 'This double-blind, placebo-controlled study shows that inhaled thingerol, 50 g b.d., is more effective than wotsiterol, 200 mg q.i.d., in controlling the nocturnal symptoms of asthma.'

▲ Answer subsidiary questions in order of importance

If there is more than one question to be answered, answer them in order of importance – for example, primary outcome measures before secondary outcome measures, efficacy before side-effects.

▲ Go on to support the answer using your own results and those of others

Do not repeat your results in detail. Simply give selected data in order to back up the general points that you make. When supporting the answer, again organize the topics from the most important to the least important.

▲ Then explain how the answer fits in (or does not fit in) with other published results

Again, you should address topics in order of importance. Highlight similarities between the results of your study and other well-respected studies, but do not be afraid to draw attention to differences.

▲ Do not ignore 'inconvenient' results

It is important to explain (as far as you can) any unexpected findings, or any results that are not consistent with your answer. If you do not, the reviewer may assume that you have not noticed the problem. If you can offer no reasonable explanation for an inconsistent result, it is acceptable to say so. Do not be tempted into wild flights of fancy in order to justify an apparently inexplicable finding.

▲ Do not be afraid to defend your conclusion

If you have done a good study, you should be prepared to defend your conclusion against attack. What about others who did not get the same answers? You may be able to offer explanations for the discrepancies between your study and theirs. For example, other researchers may have used different methods or studied different populations. If justified, you can highlight shortcomings in their studies compared to your own (see below).

▲ Be respectful towards other studies

It is accepted practice to dissect the shortcomings of other studies, but please be as courteous as possible while you are doing it. Your own results will be subjected to similarly severe scrutiny by your research rivals. Furthermore, there is always the chance that the reviewer was involved in the research that you are criticizing, or is a personal friend of the researchers in question. Be scrupulously objective and polite.

▲ Explain any limitations of your methods or study design

Every study has its limitations – do not be afraid to address yours. It is better for you to note limitations rather than lead the reviewer to believe that you simply have not noticed them. The CONSORT statement for reporting clinical trials specifies that limitations should be included, and some journals now have a specific subheading for limitations.

▲ Finish your discussion by restating the conclusion …

In longer discussions it is conventional to briefly restate the answer at the end, sometimes in a separate section headed 'Conclusions'. Although repetitious, this can be helpful. The last paragraph is, after all, where many readers will look to find the 'bottom line' of the study. Use a different form of words from that with which you began the discussion, to make it more interesting for the reader. In a short discussion (half a page or less), there may be no need to restate the conclusion.

▲ ... And any important implications

If your study is new or particularly important, it is acceptable to say so, using modest language. If your study has implications for future research or for clinical practice, it is also appropriate to describe these at the end of the discussion. However, if you have nothing particularly interesting to say about the implications of the study then stop after restating the answer. Conclusions that say 'further research is necessary' tend to sound a bit lame. Further research is *always* necessary in science.

▲ Be careful with tenses

It is likely that you will use a mixture of past and present tenses in the discussion. You should use the present tense for the answer. Use the past tense for your results and those of others, but present tense for established fact. For example, you could say: 'Smith *et al. found* that X was associated with Y, but our results suggest that this *is* not the case. We *found* that X *was* correlated only with Z'.

▲ Choose your 'proving' words carefully according to strength

'Prove' is the strongest word we can use about our findings, but it can rarely be used in biomedical studies. Here are some others, in descending order of strength. Think about which one matches the strength of your conclusions. Can you think of any others?

> show
> demonstrate
> indicate
> suggest
> imply.

▲ Be cautious ...

Very little is incontrovertible in science. It is accepted and appropriate to use qualifying words such as:

> may be
> might be

> could be
> probably
> possibly

▲ ... But not excessively so

However, do not qualify so much that you show little confidence in your results.

- 'These results suggest that the cause of X is Y' is acceptable.
- 'These results suggest that the cause of X may be Y' is weaker, but may be appropriate if you are being very cautious.
- 'These results suggest the possibility that the cause of X may ultimately be determined to be Y' is ridiculously overcautious.

▲ Make the logic of your argument clear to the reader

Use 'signalling' words to underline the logic of your argument. For example:

> This study shows …
> The evidence is that …
> For example, …
> Contrary to our expectation, …
> Surprisingly, …
> To summarize, …
> In conclusion, …

▲ In a very long discussion subheadings may be helpful

In very long papers, in which results fall into several categories that must be discussed separately, some journals will allow the use of subheadings. However, in a typical original research paper, the discussion should not be so long that subheadings are necessary.

▲ Save some of your references for the discussion – do not put them all in the introduction

There is a temptation to mention all the relevant references in the introduction. This can leave you with the feeling that you have nothing new to say when you get to the disussion. In fact, only the references that are relevant to understanding the *question* should go in the introduction. The references that are relevant to understanding the *answer* should go in the discussion. Some are, of course, relevant to both. Since the references relevant to the answer are more important than the general background, the discussion is likely to be longer than the introduction. Readers are more interested in the results of your study than in generalizations.

▲ If using the author–year system, minimize repetition of authors' names in the text

If the references in your paper are according to the author–year system, there is no need to repeat the authors' names in the main text. For example: 'Several studies have shown an association between X and Y (Smith 1987, Brown 1991, Dupree 1995)' is preferable to 'Smith, Brown and Dupree have shown an association between X and Y (Smith 1987, Brown 1991, Dupree 1995)', as it avoids unnecessary repetition.

▲ If using numbered references, mention authors' names in the text only very selectively

If you are using numbered references, there is still no need to mention the names of all the authors to whose studies you are referring unless you specifically want to link the author with the results. Thus it is perfectly acceptable to say 'Several studies have shown an association between X and Y[15–17]' but you might sometimes want to say 'Our results differ from those of Brown,[16] who found that …'

▲ Apply this reviewer's checklist to your discussion

Is the discussion:

- ❏ logical and succinct?
- ❏ well referenced (not too many)?
- ❏ accurate and fair regarding other studies' findings?
- ❏ an interpretation rather than a restatement of the results?
- ❏ free of far-fetched hypotheses?
- ❏ free of vague or unsubstantiated statements?
- ❏ frank in acknowledging limitations?
- ❏ able to explain most anomalies?

16

References

Whether you are writing a thesis, an original research paper or a review article, you will need a list of references. Typing and organizing these references can be a major chore, but fortunately there are a number of techniques you can use to make things easier. Here are some tips on dealing with references as efficiently as possible.

▲ Use reference management software

If you have to work with references all the time, as most scientists do, you will find that reference management software removes a lot of the drudgery. This software allows you to enter the various parts of each reference into a standard form, creating a permanent database. You can then paste temporary citations from this database into your word processing program, in such a way that they will be automatically formatted into a correctly-ordered reference list at the end. You can specify that they be formatted into any one of a wide range of journal styles, or even program your own. If you add or delete a reference or move chunks of text around, the programme will take care of reordering the references. Reference management software is discussed in more detail in Chapter 31. Examples include EndNote and Reference Manager.

▲ Format references correctly according to guidelines

All journals will have a standard format for references that will be described in the Instructions to Authors. For a thesis there will normally also be rules laid down by your institution. If the references in a journal article are not in the correct format, you run the risk of having the article sent back to you for amendment before the editor will look at it.

▲ Make sure you understand the instructions regarding each part of the reference ...

For example, there will be instructions for:

- how many authors to list
- whether you include the title of the paper
- whether you can abbreviate the journal title
- where you put the dates
- whether you give the journal part number
- how you cite the page range
- how you punctuate the reference
- whether certain parts are in **bold** or *italic* type.

▲ ... And how to cite it in the text

The commonest ways of citing references are:

- *Numbered.* 'As various authors have shown [1,2] ...' or 'As various authors have shown,[3-7]'. The reference list at the end is in numerical order. Check to see whether superscript numbers or brackets are to be used. Usually it is best to put reference numbers at the end of the sentence to which they refer. When superscript reference numbers are used, they go after the full stop, whereas numbers in brackets go before the full stop.
- *Author–date.* 'As has been shown (Smith & Jones, 1985)'. The reference list is in alphabetical order. Check to see how the authors are cited in the text – for example, whether you use 'and' or '&', how you use *et al.* and whether you put a comma before the date.
- *Alphabetic–numeric.* You may still come across this rather odd system in which the references are numbered in the text but the reference list is given in alphabetical order.

▲ Become familiar with the Vancouver style

The commonest format for references nowadays is the Vancouver style (see the Uniform Requirements in Appendix 1):

- *For journals*: MacIntyre PB, Pemberton JH. Pathophysiology of colonic motility disorders. *Surg Clin North Am* 1993; **73**: 1225–43.
- *For books*: Burks TF. Actions of pharmacological agents on gastrointestinal function. In: Kumar D, Wingate D, eds. *An illustrated guide to gastrointestinal motility.* London: Churchill Communications Europe, 1993: 144–61.

However, do not assume that you can always use this style – some journals use different formats.

▲ Check how many authors' names your journal requires you to give

Some journals require you to give all the authors for each reference. Others will instruct you that when a reference has six or more authors (sometimes five or more), you should give only the first three, and replace the remaining names with *et al*. If you are using reference management software, enter all the authors' names into the database whether you need them or not at the time. If you download the reference from a database this will happen automatically. Then, if you ever have to reformat the references for a journal that gives all names, they will be in the database and you will not have to go looking for them.

▲ Be thoughtful about how many references you give

In a thesis it is appropriate to give a large number of references to show that you have read all the relevant literature on the subject. However, in an original research paper you are not trying to show how well read you are. You should only give those references that are immediately relevant to the reader's understanding of the paper. A medium-sized research paper in the biomedical sciences will probably have no more than about 20–30 references. Short papers will have fewer. Long papers may have more. Some journals will tell you how many references are acceptable in the Instructions to Authors. Review articles typically have many references – after all, they are a review of the literature and do need to be comprehensive.

▲ Prefer recent references unless there is a good reason

References should be relevant and recent (except in historical reviews or where there are no recent references). Well-conducted studies are to be preferred to poorly conducted studies.

▲ Prefer references that the reader will be able to obtain

You should also choose references that will be available to the normal reader. In general, this means you should prefer journal articles. Theses, conference abstracts and unpublished conference proceedings may be more difficult to obtain and therefore should only be used when there is no better way of referencing the data. Books are citeable, but are often not the most up-to-date sources of information. You can cite websites, but think about whether the information is likely to be available long-term on the same site.

▲ In journal articles, you cannot cite papers that have not been accepted ...

If you really must, you can cite an unpublished, submitted paper in the text '(Smith E. Personal communication)' or 'Smith E. Unpublished data'. However, you cannot include it in the reference list. Check the Instructions to Authors to see exactly how unpublished material should be cited.

▲ ... But you can cite papers that have been accepted but not yet published

It is acceptable to cite a paper that has been accepted in the reference list like this:

Smith E. A randomized, double-blind, placebo-controlled study of the efficacy and safety of hairolol in male-pattern baldness. *Journal of Industrial Trichology*. In press 1997.

Some journals require a copy of the acceptance letter to prove that a paper cited in this way has really been accepted. Again, check the Instructions to Authors for the preferred format.

▲ Be exact when citing references

It is very frustrating for readers to send for a paper, only to find that the authors' names are wrong, there is no such paper in that journal or the page range is wrong. One survey showed that as many as 4 out of 10 references had something wrong with them. So check your references carefully against the original paper. Do not assume that because you copied them from a published paper they will be right (see below).

▲ Always obtain original references for every paper you cite

It is tempting to take the word of other authors regarding the content of well-known papers in your field. However, it is your responsibility to be sure that each paper says exactly what you say it does. Surveys have shown that many papers cited as supporting a particular point do not actually do so. Even though it may take some time and trouble, it is worth getting hold of the originals of all the papers you cite, and checking exactly what it is they say.

17

Checking your
manuscript

At last your manuscript is finished. But is it? You will need to check very carefully before you send your paper to a journal or have your thesis bound. You will almost certainly find things you want to change, from small errors of grammar or punctuation to moving, adding or deleting whole sections. A carefully prepared manuscript gives a good first impression, which will gain the attention and interest of the editor, reviewers or examiner.

The tips in this chapter are based on professional editorial techniques, and will help you to turn in a polished manuscript.

▲ Take a break between writing and checking your manuscript

To find the errors in your manuscript you need to distance yourself from it somehow. Ideally, you should put it away for a few days, then look at it again. If, as somehow always seems to happen, you are up against a deadline, at least go and do something else for a few hours.

▲ Take your time

It is impossible to check your manuscript if you are in a hurry. If you work slowly and methodically you are much more likely to find errors. A skimpy check is hardly worth the effort.

▲ Take regular breaks

Checking requires intense concentration. You simply will not be able to concentrate hard for hours at a stretch, so take regular breaks. Ten minutes break in every half hour is a good rule. Make sure you get away from your desk – move around, talk to someone, have a cup of coffee, listen to some music – anything to take your mind off letters and numbers.

▲ Do not expect to find all the errors in your own work

You will be so used to your manuscript that you will never be able to find all the mistakes. A fresh 'eye' will be enormously helpful in:

- spotting any scientific problems on which the reviewers may comment
- checking the overall structure and content from a reader's point of view
- finding small errors of English and typing mistakes.

You will be amazed at the errors that can be found by someone who is new to the manuscript.

▲ You need someone to check the science …

It is often useful to have two or more other people read your manuscript. You need at least one qualified scientist to check the scientific content and overall structure. You could call on your boss, supervisor or research colleagues.

▲ … And someone to check the English …

You also need someone to check for minor errors of English, punctuation and so on. If your scientific 'checker' is also very meticulous and good at English he can do this as he goes along. However, scientists (including native speakers) are not always good at English! Nor do they necessarily have the meticulous mind-set needed for this work. You may want to get a second 'checker', who need not necessarily be scientifically qualified. If you are lucky, your partner or a member of your family may be a good 'checker'.

▲ … but one person (you) has to take overall responsibility

If your manuscript has several authors, or has been checked by several people, there may be differences of opinion about what is the best way to write up certain ideas.

There may also be quibbles about more minor matters of writing style. In the end, someone – normally you, as first author – has to arbitrate disputes and make a final decision about disputed points.

▲ Remember that larger journals have copy-editors for accepted papers …

You can expect journal copy-editors to correct small matters of English once your paper is accepted for publication. Copy-editors can be especially helpful if you are not a native English speaker. They will also make sure your manuscript complies with the journal's house-style rules, though they will expect you to have made a good attempt at meeting the requirements set out in the Instructions to Authors. Smaller journals and many online journals have minimal copy-editing – they cannot afford it. In this case, authors need to check their submissions even more carefully.

▲ … But do not expect them always to spot mistakes in the science

Journal copy-editors cannot, however, be expected to find errors such as the wrong numbers given for your results, or statements that do not say what you meant to say. In practice they are very good at spotting inconsistencies and raising queries, but every such query causes an infinitesimal delay in the progress of your paper towards publication.

▲ Do not try to check every aspect of your manuscript in one reading

Several 'passes' through your manuscript are usually necessary – you will find more mistakes if you concentrate on one thing at a time. Some passes may take some time, others can be accomplished very quickly. You can work at your own way of doing this. I would normally do separate passes for:

- general impression – structure, suitability
- completeness
- headings
- figures and tables
- references
- journal style
- spelling, grammar etc.

▲ Use a checklist

You will be less likely to miss errors if you check systematically, using a checklist. An example is given in Appendix 2, but you may want to draw up your own.

▲ Get a different perspective

You may find it easier to detect mistakes in a manuscript that looks different from the way you are used to seeing it. If you have been reading it on the computer screen, try printing it out. If you are used to seeing it on white paper, try printing it out on different coloured paper or use a different font (e.g. Ariel instead of Times).

▲ Try checking spelling and grammar line by line

It may help you to concentrate on small details of spelling and grammar if you use a ruler or piece of paper placed over the page. This will help you focus on one line at a time.

▲ Use your spell checker carefully

The spell checker on your word processor is very helpful, but it will not find all errors. For example if you write 'two' as 'tow', it will not be able to tell the difference, because 'tow' is also a word. In addition, there will be many scientific words that are not in the spell checker's dictionary. If you add such words to the dictionary as you encounter them, this will speed up spell-checking in the long term. You can also use a specialized spell checker, such as *Stedman's Medical Dictionary*, which can be integrated into your word processor (see Chapter 31).

▲ Do not expect too much from your grammar checker

Well-known word-processing programmes like Word and WordPerfect come with a built-in grammar checker. These are getting better all the time, but at the moment are not good enough to pick up all the grammatical errors in your manuscript. Moreover, they will sometimes tell you there is a problem where none exists. They are interesting to use as a learning exercise, but there is no substitute at present for human intelligence. If your grammar is not very good, then try to get someone with more expertise to read your manuscript.

18

Research papers and reviews: submitting your manuscript

When you submit a paper to a journal, you will send it with an electronic submission form or a covering email. There is usually space in a submission form to write a short covering note. Because the submission is the first thing the editor sees, it plays an important part in creating a good first impression for your paper. A carefully written covering note can have a small, but important, effect in increasing your chances of publication. A carelessly written covering note might even result in your paper failing to receive the consideration it deserves.

▲ Include all essential components of the submission form

You may be required to complete:

❏ the title of the journal (for publishers that publish multiple journals)
❏ the name, address, phone, fax and e-mail numbers of the submitting author
❏ the name, address, phone, fax and e-mail numbers of the author to whom correspondence should be addressed (if different from the submitting author)
❏ the title of the paper
❏ whether the paper falls into a particular category (e.g. short communication, review article) or section of the journal
❏ the names of all the authors

❑ an appropriate statement that the content of the paper has not been published elsewhere, nor is it currently under consideration by another journal
❑ whether you are willing to pay any charges that may be relevant (e.g. the cost of colour illustrations or for immediate open access)
❑ the signatures of all the authors (see below).

▲ Consider these additional optional components

Depending on the circumstances, you may also wish to include the following:

❑ a few words about the content of the paper (see below)
❑ a brief note on why you selected the journal
❑ a statement regarding optional or online components (e.g. colour photographs, detailed methods)
❑ a note of any material submitted that is for information rather than publication (i.e. tabulated data to back up graphs)
❑ suggestions for reviewers (see below)
❑ any conditions on publication (try to make these as few as possible)
❑ any restrictions on copyright transfer (see below).

▲ It is sometimes helpful to say why you selected the journal

Often it will be obvious why you chose the journal – for example, it may simply be the best in its field. There is no need to try to flatter the editor by saying so – that would be embarrassing and artificial. Sometimes, however, the editor may be a little surprised by your choice of journal if the paper is somewhat outside its usual remit. For example, if you submit a paper on molecular biology to a general clinical journal, it would be appropriate to point out that you believe your results have important implications for clinical medicine.

▲ You can draw attention to key features of your paper – but be brief

It is acceptable to draw the editor's attention to any features of your paper that readers are likely to find interesting. This may be genuinely helpful to a busy editor.

However, be very careful not to overstate your case. Just one or two modestly worded sentences will be enough. Editors do not like to feel that you are trying to 'sell' your paper like a used car.

Something like this might be appropriate:

As far as we are aware, this study is the first placebo-controlled trial to show a therapeutic effect of camomile tea in tension headache. It was conducted as a result of our questionnaire survey among camomile users, reported as a Short Communication in your journal last year (*Eur J Med Bot* 1996; **24**: 36–7).

We believe that this topic will be of interest to your readers, as the European Society for Headache Research has recently highlighted the need for new treatments in this increasingly prevalent condition.

The paper includes five figures and an additional three figures for inclusion as supplementary information …

▲ Make sure you address the issues of repetitive publication …

It is important to state that the content of your paper has not been published elsewhere. If any part of your paper *has* been published elsewhere, and for some reason you consider that repetitive publication is justified, you need to explain why. For example, if your paper was previously published in another language in a local journal, you will need to explain that you consider publication in English in an international journal important, in order to make the data available to a wider audience.

▲ … And duplicate submission

A paper can only be sent to one journal at a time. You cannot send your paper to two journals at once in the hope of accelerating the publication process. Editors are unwilling to spend time on papers if there is a danger of them being subsequently withdrawn because of acceptance elsewhere. After all, no one likes to be second choice. The submission form often asks you to confirm that your paper is not currently under consideration by any other journal.

▲ If you will not be able to transfer copyright to the journal, say so

Most journals (except online-only journals) expect that you will sign over copyright of your paper to them when it is accepted. If for any reason you cannot do this (e.g. because your employer does not permit it), you should say so in the covering letter.

▲ There is usually no need to give the paper's rejection history

If your paper has already been rejected by another journal (or journals) there is usually no need to say so. However, a few journals may request information on previous submissions and copies of any previous reviewers' comments. It is important to reformat your paper in line with the new journal's Instructions to Authors. Editors become easily annoyed, if, for example, the references have clearly been formatted for another publication.

▲ It is often helpful to suggest one or more reviewers

Although journals maintain databases of reviewers, the editor will often be open to suggestions from authors, and some specifically request them. In fact, in very specialized areas, the author is often the best person to identify a suitable expert to comment on the paper. If you suggest one or more reviewers, it is appropriate to add that they have not been involved in the study or the preparation of the paper.

▲ If you really must, you can ask that certain reviewers be avoided

There may be some circumstances in which you are anxious that a particular person should not review your paper. For example, you may feel that a rival research group should not have access to your results before publication. Or you may feel that a certain reviewer is unduly prejudiced and will not give your paper a fair chance.

You have the right to ask the editor not to send your paper to certain specified individuals, but you must be prepared to withdraw if the editor is not happy with this arrangement. 'I would prefer that my paper not be reviewed by Dr X of the University of Y. If you are unable to meet this request, I would rather withdraw my paper from submission to this journal.' Although requesting that one or two reviewers be avoided is acceptable, a long list is unreasonable and makes you look paranoid.

▲ Tell the editor if any of the contents of the submission are provided for information only …

Some journals request the original data from which graphs are plotted. This is for the benefit of the reviewers who will assess the paper. If you have included such material, it is important to say so, and to distinguish it clearly from the paper itself.

▲ ... Or for optional publication

If you would like the journal to publish all of your manuscript, but would be willing for it to miss out certain parts (e.g. large tables, detailed methods, photographs), explain this in the letter. Some journals will be willing to put this supplementary data online.

▲ Note that the address for correspondence may not be the same as that of the first author

Do not leave the editor to assume that correspondence should automatically be addressed to the first author at the same address as that given on the paper. There are many circumstances in which this is not the case. For example, the first author may have moved to another institution and will want to receive correspondence at his or her new address; or the first author may have retired, and another of the authors may be taking over responsibility for progressing the paper to publication.

▲ Check you have included everything

When you are ready to submit your manuscript, check that you have included:

❏ submission form
❏ all files required for text, figures, tables
❏ copies of permission letters from patients or guardians, if required
❏ copies of permission letters from other journals to reproduce figures, if required
❏ copies of permission letters to quote unpublished data, if required.

19

Dealing with the editor's and reviewers' comments

Let us imagine that you have submitted your paper to a journal, and it has been returned to you with the editor's and reviewers' comments. How you are feeling now will depend on whether you have been told that your paper has been:

- rejected outright as unsuitable for that journal
- rejected, with an invitation to resubmit if certain amendments can be made
- accepted, subject to minor revisions.

If your paper has been accepted, congratulations! If not, here are some suggestions on what to do next.

▲ Remember that the editor's decision is final

If the editor rejects your paper outright, with no hope for resubmission, there is nothing you can do. Often, the reason given will be that your paper 'does not fit within the journal's current remit' or something similar. You may sometimes find this explanation rather thin, especially if you have seen the journal publish other papers on the same subject. However, it may be that the editor has accepted too many papers on this subject already, and is looking for something different. Or it may be a diplomatic way of saying 'not interesting enough for us'. In any event, you have no option but to send your paper elsewhere.

▲ Look carefully at why your paper has been rejected

Whether you decide to revise and resubmit your paper to the same journal or give up and go elsewhere depends on why it was rejected and if it is practical to correct the problem. The commonest reasons for rejection, other than unsuitability for the journal, are:

- problems with experimental design
- problems with statistical analysis
- omissions in reporting
- errors of inference (i.e. a poor discussion).

▲ Revise and resubmit your paper to the same journal if the problem can easily be corrected

It makes sense to revise your paper and resubmit it to the same journal if:

- it was rejected mainly because it was too long
- missing data can be added
- misinterpretation of the data can be corrected
- the data can be re-analysed to improve the statistics
- additional research can be done without too much difficulty
- the editor or reviewers made encouraging comments.

▲ Revise and resubmit your paper elsewhere if the problem is beyond correction

If your paper is rejected on the grounds of study design, or other irrevocable errors, you can still submit it elsewhere. If you choose another journal that does not set such stringent standards, you may be fortunate enough to get it published in spite of its defects.

▲ Remember you do not have to agree with all the reviewers' comments

It is very unwise to argue aggressively with the reviewers. However, if you genuinely feel that they have misunderstood or misinterpreted your paper, it is acceptable to write to the editor, stating your point of view. However, unless you are very convinced that you are right, and very determined to get published in that particular journal, you are likely to find that entering into a protracted correspondence is not worthwhile.

▲ Watch out for disagreements between reviewers

You may find that the the reviewers (usually there are two) do not agree with each other. Usually, the editor will act as arbitrator. If the editor has not already addressed any disagreement, and simply sends you the two conflicting sets of comments, it is usually a good idea to write back, stating your own point of view and asking for the editor's advice.

▲ Have a contingency plan ready

However confident you are, you should always be prepared for the possibility of a rejection that cannot be salvaged. It pays to have a second choice of journal in mind, and a copy of the Instructions to Authors at the ready. Then, if your paper is rejected, you will soon be ready to resubmit it elsewhere.

▲ Remember that about 80% of papers eventually get published somewhere

Rejection from your first choice of journal does not mean you should give up. If you thought your study was good enough to write up in the first place, try to have some confidence in your own judgement. You may have taken a gamble in pitching your choice of journal too high, but could still have a good chance of acceptance by another, less prestigious but still respectable, journal.

▲ If you resubmit elsewhere, make sure you revise your paper to the style of the new journal

It is very annoying for editors to receive a manuscript that has obviously been prepared for another journal. Revise your paper carefully to fit the new journal's Instructions to Authors. Remove any clues to prior rejections, such as footers that identify the paper as having been sent to a different journal.

▲ Make what use you can of the reviewers' comments, even if sending your paper to a different journal

Take due note of the comments made by the journal that rejected your paper, and do what you can to improve it. You may not be able to do anything about the study design, but you may want to defend it pre-emptively in the discussion. There may be other errors of omission or interpretation that you can easily correct.

▲ Remember these rules for how to get your paper published

Your paper is likely to be published if you:

- conduct a good study
- choose an appropriate journal
- prepare the manuscript carefully
- anticipate the reviewers' comments
- write a positive/informative covering letter
- recognize you cannot control all the factors
- have a contingency plan in case of rejection.

20

Review articles and
book chapters

All of us rely to some extent on review articles and books to keep up to date. The scientific literature is so vast that no one could possibly read everything relevant to their subject. The problem is most acute for people working in clinical medicine, who are fully stretched just seeing their patients without trying to read everything that could possibly be relevant to them. Review articles and review chapters in books therefore play an essential role in keeping clinicians and researchers up to date, and alerting us to important shifts in opinion or practice.

▲ A review article or book chapter can help get your name known

A good review article or book chapter not only benefits your fellow scientists – if you are a young scientist, it also benefits your career. It can bring your name to the attention of a much wider audience than would a single piece of original research, and helps to establish you as an expert in your field.

▲ Do not underestimate the amount of work involved

Writing a review article or book chapter is very worthwhile, provided it is approached in a systematic and objective way. But it is not usually a quick or easy task. However well you know your subject, it is a mistake to think that a review article or book chapter can be 'dashed off' in a few days. Generally speaking, it is considerably more difficult and time-consuming than writing an original research paper.

▲ If the review is commissioned, get a good brief

Usually, a review will be commissioned by the editor of a journal or book. If you receive a letter asking you to write a review, you may well find that an outline of the proposed content is enclosed.

▲ If in doubt, ask plenty of questions

If you have not been thoroughly briefed by a commissioning letter, it is your job to ask some important questions before you start to write. For example:

- who is the intended audience?
- which topics should you include?
- which topics should you exclude?
- should you stress a particular point of view?
- how long should the review be?
- how many figures and tables are required?
- how many references would be appropriate?
- when is your deadline?

Of course, the editor may say that you have a free hand – it is up to you. But often you will find that they do have a preconceived idea of what your review should cover, and in how much detail.

▲ If other authors are involved, beware of overlap

In a multi-author book, there is often potential for overlap between the chapters. Check with the editor who else is contributing, and whether there are likely to be any areas of overlap. If so, ask how this should be managed. The editor may lay down some boundaries, or invite you to contact the other author(s) and work with them to 'carve up' the subject between you. On the other hand, some editors may take the view that more than one viewpoint on the same subject will add something useful to the book.

▲ If the review is your idea, check it out with your intended journal

Some journals only accept commissioned reviews. Others sometimes accept reviews submitted speculatively. However, it would be a big gamble to take the time and trouble required to write a good review, without knowing whether it fits in with the journal's publication policy. If you have an idea for a review, it is a good plan to telephone the editor of the journal to see whether he or she would be interested. The editor may ask you to submit a detailed outline. Of course, they are unlikely to agree definitely to publish without seeing the completed review – among the top journals, peer review is usually just as important for review articles as it is for original research papers.

▲ Decide what kind of article you are going to write

Reviews and book chapters come in many different shapes and sizes. For example, they may be:

- comprehensive – everything there is to know about a particular topic
- selective – deliberately excluding particular topics or approaches
- descriptive – simply outlining what has been done
- evaluative – highlighting 'good' studies
- argumentative – supporting one point of view against another.

▲ Decide where you are going to get your information

Many reviews and book chapters are based exclusively on material available in the 'scientific literature' – published papers, abstracts and theses. Others include un-published data from the author's own studies (sometimes used rather cynically as a way of publishing data that would not make a paper on its own).

▲ Consider whether true meta-analysis is possible ...

Some review articles are based on meta-analysis, not only reviewing the data in the literature, but combining and reanalysing it, sometimes including unpublished data. The current popularity of 'evidence-based medicine' means that such reviews are likely to be well received, but they require a lot of work and considerable statistical knowledge.

▲ ... Or whether a less statistically rigorous approach is required

Even in reviews that do not include meta-analysis, it is appropriate to show that you have looked at all the published studies, excluded those that do not meet specified criteria, and objectively assessed the implications of the rest.

▲ Search the literature carefully

For a review to be authoritative, it is important to consider all the relevant papers. To do this, you need to conduct a careful literature search. Depending on the topic, you may need to consult more than one database. You will probably find it helpful to consult a scientific information specialist in order to devise a foolproof search strategy.

▲ Get copies of all the references and read the relevant parts

As mentioned in Chapter 16, it is your responsibility to check that each reference says what you say it says. Inadvertent misrepresentation of the contents of scientific papers is quite common, and can be perpetuated from one review article to another. Make sure that this does not apply to you. You do not usually have to read all of every paper – often just the abstract will give you a good idea of the main points. Then you can read the whole of just the most relevant papers.

▲ Have a 'big idea'

Every piece of writing should have a 'big idea'. Nowhere is this more important than in a review. Sometimes your idea may be very big, e.g. 'Everything known about the causes, diagnosis and treatment of X'. More often, however, it will be something more specific, e.g. 'Based on the available evidence, the best way of treating X in elderly patients is the ABC method'. If you cannot write your big idea down in a single sentence, you are not ready to start writing the article.

▲ Draw up a detailed plan

Planning is all-important when writing long and complex documents. If you are working to a detailed outline, you will be confident that you are not missing out essential parts of your argument or story. You will also be able to draw up a time-table ensuring that you meet your deadline. Surprise your publisher by being one of the few authors who send their manuscripts in on time! To draw up your plan, try the techniques listed in Chapter 5.

▲ Try writing a card or sticky note for each reference ...

The 'yellow sticky' technique described in Chapter 5 is particularly useful for review articles. To recap, you write one or more sticky notes or file cards for each reference, and arrange them in a logical order to create the plan for your article.

▲ ... Or photocopy just the top half of each first page ...

An alternative to the 'yellow sticky' technique is to photocopy just the top half of the front page of each paper. This enables you to reduce the amount of paper you have to deal with, and allows you to arrange references in logical groups. (Thanks to Liz Wager of Janssen-Cilag for introducing me to this tip.)

▲ ... Or just arrange the references in folders by topic

You can also arrange your references in folders (or piles on the floor) by topic. One disadvantage of this is that some references may come under more than one heading and you therefore want to put them in more than one file. You can, of course, overcome this by combining the 'files' and 'yellow sticky' techniques, and just write cards or sticky notes for those references you want to have in two files at once. A second disadvantage is that files are physically unwieldy – unlike sticky notes, it is hard to spread all the references out and see the whole picture at once.

▲ Use standard structures where appropriate

Some review articles have standardized structures. For example, if you were writing a comprehensive review of a new drug, it might follow this sort of structure:

- the disease area
- previous treatments
- chemistry
- pharmacology
- pharmacokinetics
- toxicology
- animal models of disease
- dose-ranging studies
- efficacy in humans (vs placebo and vs comparators)
- adverse effects in humans
- conclusions and recommendations.

▲ Include a statement of how you got your information

Nowadays, it is customary to give some information in your review about how you obtained the references, e.g. 'We searched MedLine and Embase for English-language papers published between 1917 and 1997, using the search terms …'

▲ Think carefully about which studies you include

To paraphrase George Orwell, all studies are equal, but some are more equal than others. Usually, you will want to ascribe more weight to the 'best' studies. You may decide not to mention seriously flawed studies at all, or to mention them but not discuss them in detail. Just as you would describe how you selected subjects or patients for an experiment, you should include inclusion and exclusion criteria for papers in your review. For example, did you only evaluate blinded studies, or did you include open studies as well? Why?

▲ Within sections and paragraphs, double-check for logical order

Readers expect to see logical order in your writing. Note that you may need to use different kinds of logical order in different parts of your review. For example:

- chronological – early studies to recent studies
- order of importance – best studies first, minor studies last
- structural – by body system or geographical area
- deductive – e.g. saturated fat is bad for us, sausages are full of saturated fat, therefore we should avoid eating sausages.

▲ Structure your arguments carefully

Still on the subject of logic, remember that readers must be able to follow the development after your argument. Make sure that every statement you make is supported by the evidence. Never assume that it is obvious. You also need to make sure that readers do not lose sight of the argument – a summary sentence or paragraph every now and then is a good idea.

▲ Prepare yourself for peer review

Even if your review is commissioned, it may still be subject to peer review. Here is a checklist of criteria used to examine review articles:

- ❏ was the purpose of the review stated?
- ❏ how was the literature selected?
- ❏ how were the articles assessed?
- ❏ were differences in study findings analysed and explained?
- ❏ were studies grouped appropriately?
- ❏ were the conclusions supported by data?
- ❏ were directions for future research specified?

▲ Write an informative abstract or summary, if the format allows

For readers, an abstract or summary that outlines the main points of the article or chapter is very useful. When a review-article title is downloaded from an on-line database, searchers tend to feel cheated if they do not find an abstract attached. So, assuming that the format of the journal or book allows it, provide an informative abstract or summary. Try to avoid the sort of summary that says 'Recommendations are made for approaches to …' This leaves readers still wondering what the recommendations are.

It is harder to write an informative summary of a long article, but very worthwhile.

21

Theses and dissertations

Although there is a lot more to postgraduate research than writing, your thesis or dissertation is undoubtedly the end-product. Your examiners will use it to judge the quality of your research – since they could not be there watching you, it is all they have to go on.

For many people, the writing of the thesis is a more daunting prospect than all the rest of the research put together. Yet, writing a thesis need not be such a Herculean task if you follow these common-sense tips. (Note: the term 'thesis' is used here to cover both theses and dissertations.)

▲ Check the rules and regulations before you start

Begin by obtaining and studying the regulations for your degree in your university. Most universities lay down detailed rules governing the length, organization and presentation of theses. The detail may extend to such fine points as abbreviations, reference style, margins, spacing, typeface, type of paper and binding. Failure to follow these regulations could result in a delay in your thesis being examined.

▲ Start writing early

It is usually best to start work on your thesis as early as possible. While it may be tempting to wait until all your experimental work is completed, this is rarely practical. It is preferable to write up individual experiments as you complete them. You can then amalgamate sections as appropriate when you get to the completion phase of your thesis. In any case, you will probably want to write papers for publication as your research progresses. You may also be required to submit regular progress reports.

▲ Use a computerized reference management system from day one

As described in Chapter 31, with reference management software you only ever have to type a reference once – or maybe not at all, if you download it from a database. Using one of these systems from the very first day of your research programme will make your life immeasurably easier, and greatly speed the writing of your thesis.

▲ Be organized about storage of data, references and manuscripts

Writing your thesis will be much easier if you have swift access to everything you need. This applies to your raw data, references and previous draft manuscripts. Work out a system for storing your references, whether as paper copies or as pdf files on your computer. Reference management programs allow you to link your database entries to pdf files.

▲ Use 'downtime' to do some writing

There will be times when you are not able to get on with the practical side of your research. Perhaps you are waiting for an experiment to finish; maybe your equipment is out of service; or maybe you are simply stuck for what to do next. You can use these 'downtimes' to write up your methods, results of completed experiments or parts of your introduction.

▲ Plan carefully

As said elsewhere in this book, planning is the foundation of effective writing. Planning your thesis is a formidable task. Yet, you can apply exactly the same rules to your thesis as you would to other major writing projects. Try approaches such as mind-mapping and the 'yellow sticky' technique (see Chapter 5).

▲ Set a page budget and interim deadlines

As described in Chapter 5, for any big piece of writing, it is important to decide in advance approximately how long each section should be. You do not want to spend many hours polishing your introduction, only to find that it is far too long relative to the length of your other sections. You should also budget your time, so that you know you will be able to complete the writing painlessly in the hours, days or weeks available. For more information on setting page budgets and managing your time, see Chapters 5 and 29.

▲ Decide on whether the 'big paper' or 'mini-papers' approach is appropriate

There are two main approaches to writing a thesis based on experimental work:

1 like a single, gigantic paper, organized into the introduction, methods, results and discussion
2 like a series of papers, with a global introduction and discussion drawing them all together.

Which you choose will depend on the type of research you have done, and the regulations of your university.

▲ Look at other theses for ideas

It can be helpful to look at other people's theses, especially those from your own department. Choose examples that you know were well received by the examiners. You can glean many useful ideas on organization, layout and illustrations. However, be sure that any bright ideas you borrow from other theses meet the statutory requirements of your university.

▲ Finish writing early

If starting writing early is a good idea, finishing early is an even better idea. You will need the remaining time to revise your draft, seek comments from your supervisor and colleagues, incorporate those comments, proofread your thesis, check references, get illustrations prepared and finally have your thesis printed and bound. You may even need to do some additional experimental work or statistical analyses to fill in any gaps that you noticed when writing up your results.

▲ Get your supervisor's input early

Once you have developed a plan for your thesis, check it out with your supervisor. Then, get your supervisor's comments on each section as soon as it is completed. Finally, ask your supervisor to read through the whole thesis to make sure it hangs together. Obtaining comments in easy stages will:

- make sure that you have time to take advantage of any suggestions your supervisor may make regarding content, organization or presentation
- improve the quality of your supervisor's comments – the more time you allow, the more detailed and carefully considered their comments will be.

▲ Prepare your figures in easy stages

You will probably have many graphs and charts in your thesis, and possibly photographs or other illustrations. It is a good idea to prepare these as you go along, to save a rush at the last minute. Even though preparing illustrations is now much faster than it was in the days of pen and ink, computer-generated illustrations still take time to perfect.

▲ Make sure you use a standard style for figures and tables

You should decide early on a standard style for details such as axes labels, units, abbreviations etc. in figures and tables. Write down this style and stick to it. Check that it is compatible with university regulations.

▲ Be obsessed with backups

When writing a thesis, your data are your most precious possession. Your second most precious possession is any writing in progress or completed. Make sure that you have up-to-date backups of both in case of disaster. Have backups stored in at least two places. That way, if the university or your home goes up in flames, or your computer is stolen, all is not lost.

▲ Give your abstract and introduction an extra polish

The abstract and introduction are the first parts of your thesis the examiners will read. These parts of the thesis set the tone for everything that is to come. Just as a person makes an indelible impression on you in the first 30 seconds, a good abstract can 'sell' your thesis, whereas a bad one can put examiners off. Although examiners will conscientiously read every bit of your thesis, it is very hard to wipe out these first impressions. So make sure your thesis gives an excellent impression, starting on the first page.

▲ Ask a friend to help with proofreading

As discussed in Chapter 17, it is impossible to find all the mistakes in your own work – you are just too close to it. Your supervisor will probably also find it difficult to spot mistakes in something so familiar, and is in any case more concerned with the sci- entific content. You need a another 'eye' – perhaps a colleague or fellow student with a good eye for detail. Or you could press a partner or friend into service. You could offer a reward – perhaps a celebratory meal on completion of the thesis. Or you could simply offer to reciprocate by proofreading their thesis when the time comes.

▲ Never trust hardware

Your word-processing and graphics programs are unlikely to let you down. Personal computers are usually fairly reliable, though networks may not be. But you would be well advised to plan for problems when it comes to printers, plotters and photo- copiers; they always seen to break down or run out of consumables when you are in a hurry.

▲ Allow plenty of time for printing, copying and binding

Allow plenty of time for printing out and photocopying your thesis. If you take it to a copy shop for copying and binding, check each photocopy before it is bound to ensure that all the pages are there. It is not unknown for pages to be missing or bound in the wrong order.

22

How to write a book

Writing a book is not very different from other kinds of scientific writing – there is just a lot more to write. You may already have some experience of contributing chapters to books or writing long reviews. You may also have written a PhD thesis, many of which are book-length. So, if you want to write a book, do not be daunted by the scale of the project. These tips will help you cut it down to a manageable size.

▲ Have a good idea

You will feel much more confident and motivated if you start with a very clear idea of what the book will be about and who will want to read it. Ask yourself:

- has this been said before?
- if so, how recently has it been said?
- have I something new to say, or a different approach?
- who would want to read this book?

If you have something new to say, or a new approach to an old subject, you are more likely to be able to sell your idea to a publisher than if you have a 'me too' idea.

▲ Be sure that you really want to do it

Writing a book will take many weeks of your valuable time, for very modest rewards. If you are doing it for the love of it, go ahead. If you are doing it to enhance your academic career, there may be easier ways of doing so.

▲ Find a publisher early

You can start looking seriously for a publisher once you have completed an outline and maybe two or three sample chapters. There is no point in waiting until you have completed the entire manuscript – at worst, you could find yourself putting in months of work on an unsaleable idea.

▲ Choose the right kind of publisher for the book you have in mind

If you take on the task of finding a publisher yourself, look carefully at the different companies that publish in your chosen area. Are they a mainstream or specialist publishers? What other books do they have on their list? Does your book appear to complement their existing list? How would they distribute your book?

▲ For non-academic books, get an agent

It is usual for authors of academic books to approach publishers direct. But if your book is for a wider audience (e.g. a book for patients or the general public), and you would like to place it with a mainstream publisher, it is best to get an agent. Publishers pay attention to book proposals submitted by agents, whereas those submitted directly by authors tend to sink to the bottom of the pile. The agent will negotiate with the publisher on your behalf, and may well be able to get you an advance against royalties. They will take a commission of about 10% – well worth it for the effort saved. You can find an agent through the *Writers' and Artists' Yearbook* (available from public libraries).

▲ Write a 'book proposal'

A book proposal is a document designed to sell your idea to a publisher. It can also help to convince an agent to take you on. A typical proposal will contain:

- a one-page synopsis describing what the book is about and what kind of readers it can be expected to attract
- a market analysis, briefly summarizing what other recently published books are available on the topic and why yours is different
- an expanded table of contents showing exactly what will be in each chapter
- two or three sample chapters, chosen to be as interesting as possible.

▲ Give yourself enough time

If you are writing the book in your 'spare' time, think how long you will need to complete it. For a typical book of 50–70 000 words, a year of spare-time writing is probably realistic. Double that if your spare time is already very busy.

▲ Set yourself interim deadlines

You will avoid a last minute panic if you try to write a little every week, or even every day. Just think – an easy 200 words a day could result in a book in a year.

▲ Get help where you can

You do not need to go it alone – colleagues and friends will usually be flattered to be asked to review specific chapters and suggest improvements. You might even want to co-opt them as co-authors (acknowledged and recompensed as appropriate).

▲ Do not expect to make a lot of money

Unless you are lucky enough to write a best seller, or a textbook that makes it onto school syllabuses, your book is unlikely to make you rich. In non-fiction publishing, an advance of around £1000 is considered generous, and more often there is no advance at all. If you do get an advance, this will be deducted from any subsequent royalties. Royalties are 10–12% of the purchase price of the book, so you will have to sell a lot of copies before you start to make a return on your investment of time and energy. Nevertheless, having a book published can have many non-financial benefits. In addition to the personal satisfaction it gives you, it can enhance your credibility as a scientist and communicator.

▲ Once your book is published, help sales in any way you can

Your publishers will make their own efforts to maximize sales of your book – for example, by sending out review copies. However, you can help to increase sales yourself. For instance, you can write related articles for the popular or professional press, give talks and get yourself interviewed by the newspapers or radio.

23

Informal science writing

Not all scientific articles have to be written for peer-reviewed journals. There are many opportunities to write articles for journals, magazines and newsletters, perhaps communicating with a wider audience. We will call these 'informal' articles, though in practice their formality varies widely according to the publication. They can be aimed at a wide range of audiences, including the lay public, and can be great fun to write. While not adding the same lustre to your publications list as a peer-reviewed article, informal articles help to get your name and your research better known.

▲ Get a commission or check out your idea first

You may be commissioned to write such an article by the editor of the publication. Or you may have a good idea – in which case it is wise to write or telephone first to check whether your contribution would be appreciated. Magazine or newsletter editors are likely to be cautious about undertaking to publish an article they have never seen, but will usually tell you honestly about what they think of your suggestion. That way, you can tailor your article to suit their readers.

▲ Write to suit your readers – not yourself

The first rule of any kind of factual writing is to write to meet your audience's needs. You do this when you write to meet demands of scientific journals for clarity, brevity and scientific accuracy. Writing to meet your audience's needs is even more important in informal articles. No one has to read an article in a magazine or newsletter – they read because they want to. Your article has to meet the 'what's in it for me' criterion.

▲ Know your readers

If you are writing for your fellow clinicians or researchers, you may already have a fairly clear idea of your readers' interests, likes and dislikes. Often, however, informal articles will be written for people with a different background, knowledge and interests from your own. For example, if you are a molecular biologist, you could find yourself explaining the clinical implications of your work to doctors, or trying to interpret them for the lay public. Before you even begin to plan your article, ask yourself:

- what are my readers interested in?
- why should they be interested in what I have to say?
- what do my readers know already?
- what information is essential in order to understand the 'big idea'?
- what information is peripheral ('nice to know' versus 'need to know')?
- what terminology will be familiar to my readers?
- what terminology will put them off?
- what do I want my readers to think, feel, decide or do as a result of reading this article?

Only when you have put yourself in your readers' shoes and answered these questions will you be ready to start writing.

▲ Get the basics right

All the rules for clear, concise, accurate writing, listed in Chapters 24–27, apply to informal science writing just as much as to formal papers and reviews. In informal writing, it is even more important to make your prose easy to read, because readers who become tired or confused can easily stop reading and look elsewhere for their information or entertainment.

▲ Pitch your article at the right level

Think carefully about the technology and concepts that your readers will be used to. Even scientific audiences may not know the technical words used in areas outside their expertise. The general public will certainly not be familiar with many scientific terms. Thus, for lay people you would usually write about 'high blood pressure' instead of 'hypertension'. On the other hand, lay people may be very knowledgeable in certain areas; for example, the parents of children with asthma probably already know quite a lot about the condition and some of the terminology used. It all comes down to knowing your audience.

▲ Say something new

People will always be more interested in your article if it tells them something they do not already know. Articles describing recent scientific discoveries are likely to attract more attention than those restating well-known facts. The topic does not have to be brand new, however. It only has to be new to your audience, or a new angle on a familiar topic.

▲ Find the conflict

People are always interested in reading about conflict. This applies not only to conflict between individuals or groups (the race to put a man on the Moon), but to conflict between ideas, between man and disease, or science and ignorance. Finding and emphasizing the conflict in your story can add interest to informal articles.

▲ Look for the human interest

People are often at least as interested in the human protagonists in a story as they are in the story itself. Thus, when describing a Nobel Prize-winning discovery, talk about the person who won the prize, as well as about the science.

▲ Add quotes for interest and endorsement

Read any news story and you will see that direct quotes are used liberally throughout. Quotes demonstrate very clearly how the person speaking feels about the subject. '"Over my dead body – I'll fight it to the last," said Dr Jones' is a far more convincing demonstration of Dr Jones's feelings than if the journalist just wrote 'Dr Jones disapproves of the proposed hospital closure'. Remember that you can quote not only things people have said, but things they have written – for example, in a presentation or scientific paper.

▲ Separate 'nice to know' from 'need to know'

Some information in your article may be useful but not essential. For example, some readers may need background information, while others may not. You can get around this situation by separating out 'nice to know' information in a box or other clearly-defined area on the page. This means that the logical flow of the main article is not disrupted. You will often see this done in popular science magazines like *New Scientist*. For example, in an article about the medical applications of growth factors, you might include a box showing how growth factors are cloned and produced in usable quantities.

▲ Put your best strawberries at the top of the basket

Lord Beaverbrook, the newspaper tycoon, advised journalists to 'put your best strawberries at the top of the basket'. In other words, do not save your conclusion until the end – put it at the beginning. Remember that only a minority of readers will be patient enough to read your article from beginning to end. It usually pays to dive straight in at the beginning with your main conclusion, then support it with the evidence. Nowhere is this more true than in news stories (see below).

▲ For news items, follow the standard structure

If you want to write an article describing recent events, follow the standard news story structure, used by journalists everywhere:

- *Headline*. A short, active statement of what happened, in the present tense, e.g. 'Oldalol cures Alzheimer's'
- *Intro*. The whole story captured in just one or two sentences, e.g. 'Oldalol can arrest or reverse the progression of Alzheimer's disease, according to a study published in the *Lancet* today. A single daily dose improves mental performance by at least 50%'
- *Facts*. More details of the story in descending order of importance, e.g. 'Researchers at the State University of Oldsville in Kentucky, USA treated more than 500 nursing-home residents with oldalol for one year. Another group received placebo treatment. After just three months, tests of short-term memory showed a marked improvement in the oldalol group, compared with a slight decline in the placebo group'
- *Background*. 'Nice to know' rather than 'need to know' information comes at the end of the story, e.g. 'Alzheimer's disease affects more than one in ten people over the age of 75'
- *Quotes*. Spread throughout to add interest, e.g. 'The leader of the research team, Professor Harold Higgins (aged 74) said "This is the biggest breakthrough since tacrine"'
- *No conclusion*. In a news story, the conclusion comes at the beginning, not at the end. Journalists realize that most readers will not make it to the end of the story.

▲ Be generous with headings and lists

In informal articles, you have a much wider choice of headings and lists than in the IMRAD structure (information, methods, results and discussion) of a scientific paper. Use headings generously to help your readers find their way around. Bullet-point lists will also act as signposts to important information.

▲ Make headings and subheadings informative

Remember that headings in informal articles can be more informative than those in a scientific paper. For example, whereas in a formal article describing a study you would have the heading 'Methods', in an informal article this could become 'At last – a model for migraine'.

▲ Be generous with illustrations

Most informal articles benefit from having plenty of illustrations. Any figures or tables previously used in scientific papers should be simplified to suit the audience of the informal publication. In contrast to scientific papers, informal articles can use illustrations simply because they are interesting or attractive. So if you have a nice photograph of your experiment in action, this is the place to use it. Many journals also have access to picture libraries, so if you do not have a suitable picture yourself you can suggest one and ask if they can obtain it. For example, if the article is about hypertension, they will probably be able to obtain a picture of a doctor measuring blood pressure.

▲ Ask rhetorical questions

In informal writing (and sometimes in formal writing), it is an accepted technique to ask questions to which you are then going to give the answer (i.e. a rhetorical question). You can use rhetorical questions in headings or in the main text of your writing. A few rhetorical questions scattered widely throughout your article can add interest, but beware of making it read like an interrogation, unless you are deliberately writing in question and answer format.

▲ Use examples and case histories

Dry technical detail can be made real by using examples, either real or invented, to suit the occasion. For example, in medical articles, both the general public and health professionals usually find patient case histories fascinating.

▲ Make statistics real

Numbers have far more impact if readers can relate them to their everyday experience. For example, you might say 'Epilepsy is common, affecting as many as one in every 130 people in the UK. This means that in a crowd of 30 000 people watching a first-division football match, over 200 may have epilepsy'.

▲ Do not give people too much to remember

Studies in the 1950s showed that most people can hold no more than seven items in their short-term memories. This means that, when giving lists of items or ideas, it is best to include no more than seven items. If you have a very long list, try to break it up into subcategories to make it more memorable. Incidentally, the most memorable number seems to be three – which is why orators and advertising copywriters continually use the rule of three (Julius Caesar: 'I came, I saw, I conquered'; advertising slogan: 'A Mars a day helps you work, rest and play').

▲ Use alliteration in moderation

Alliteration is the term used to describe the use of words beginning with the same letter or sound in close proximity (such as 'pedantic professor', or 'I came, I saw, I conquered'). You will often encounter alliteration used consciously in newspaper headlines or radio reports. We seem to have a liking for alliteration, perhaps because of the rhythm it adds to sentences. When we create neologisms in biomedicine they are often alliterations (e.g. 'big bad baby syndrome'). There is no reason why you should not use alliteration, if it comes naturally. However, try not to use it either excessively or inadvertently.

▲ Use metaphors and similes, where they help the reader

A metaphor is a figure of speech in which you say something *is* something else, e.g. 'The brain is a computer with an infinite hard disk'. A simile is a figure of speech in which you say something *is like* something else, e.g. 'Writing is like driving: we all like to think we are good at it, and are ashamed to say we are not'.

▲ Be positive

Positive writing means replacing 'It is not impossible that …' with 'It is possible that …' Similarly, avoid 'Professor Smith is not unimpressed …' and use 'Professor Smith is impressed …'

▲ Avoid unnecessary qualification

Avoiding qualification means that, wherever scientifically credible, you should write, for example, 'The experiment showed that oldalol improves cognitive function' instead of 'The experiment suggested that oldalol may improve cognitive function'. (See Chapter 15 for more information on qualification.)

24

Clear writing:
sentences

The purpose of scientific writing is to transmit information – quickly, clearly and convincingly. Common sense tells us that a well-written paper – and that means a clearly written paper – is more likely to be accepted for publication because:

- important findings will stand out and catch the editor's attention
- there is less likelihood of key points being misunderstood
- editors and reviewers are likely to feel more positive about papers that are easy to read and therefore do not waste their time.

So, here are some tips to help you write more clearly and effectively.

▲ Clear writing might help to get your paper accepted

Quality of preparation is likely to be especially important in major journals that receive thousand of papers each year, and reject as many as nine in ten of them. Good writing cannot compensate for poor research, but unclear writing can sometime obscure good research, and hence delay publication.

▲ Do not assume that because science is complex you have to write about it in a complex way

Some newcomers to scientific writing may have the impression that the 'correct' style for scientific papers is rather elaborate, using words and expressions that you would never use in everyday speech. While it is true that you will come across many papers that are written in this style, that does not mean that it is correct. Scientific writing can be formal without being elaborate or pompous. For example, there is no reason to write:

'An extensive review of the literature available at the present time leads us to the inescapable conclusion that hypertension shows a statistical association with the all too common problem of obesity.'

when you could write:

'Most studies have shown an association between obesity and hypertension'.

The second version is easier to read and has lost no essential information.

▲ Write in your natural voice

Few people are naturally convoluted or pompous in their speech, but far more adopt this style in their writing. One of the easiest ways to make your writing clearer is to write in your natural voice. How would you explain something to a scientific colleague? Good scientific writing flows naturally, like speech, only with no 'ums' or 'ers' or slang expressions, and always in a logical order.

▲ Stick to one idea per sentence

The golden rule is that a sentence should express a single thought. Often, if you write a long sentence, you will find that it contains more than one idea and can be easily split into two sentences (see below). If you have a very small thought, do not be afraid to write a short sentence.

▲ Check to see if very long sentences can be split

Ease of reading is related to two principal factors, sentence length and word length. Shortening your sentences is a simple way to make your writing easier to read. Often, you can split a long sentence into two or three shorter ones. For example:

'The efficacy and safety of grottomycin was studied in 27 patients aged 16–67 years, who had radiologically confirmed acute sinusitis with symptoms present for at least two weeks, and had not received any other antibiotics in the two weeks before the study.' (42 words)

could easily be rewritten as:

'The efficacy and safety of grottomycin was studied in 27 patients aged 16–67 years. All had radiologically confirmed acute sinusitis, with symptoms present for at least two weeks. None had received any other antibiotics in the two weeks before the study.' (14 + 14 + 13 = 41 words)

The total number of words is similar, but splitting the text into three sentences has made it easier to read. Note that you can also shorten sentences by editing out wordy and redundant phrases (see Chapter 25).

▲ Sentences of more than 30 words can usually be split

Sentence length tends to be stretched in scientific writing because we often have to include elements such as data in brackets, p values and so on. This makes it all the more important to keep sentence length within bounds. Sentences of up to 20 words are usually easiest to read. Look carefully at any sentences of more than 30 words to see if they can be shortened by editing out waste words or split into two. Do not forget that you can use short sentences – an eight-word sentence is easy to read.

▲ Vary sentence length for readability

Text that consists of nothing but long sentences is hard to read. On the other hand, text that consists only of eight-word sentences can read like machine-gun fire. The most readable combination is a mixture of short and long sentences (though that does not give you an excuse for that 45-word sentence!).

▲ If you use a long sentence, punctuate it carefully

Long sentences should be carefully punctuated to make their meaning clear. However, if your sentence has more than two commas in the middle and a full stop at the end, you can probably make it clearer by dividing it into two sentences.

▲ Use 'joining' words to clarify relationships between ideas ...

The use of 'joining' words can help the reader to see the relationships between sentences and paragraphs. Examples of 'joining' words include:

> and
> but
> however
> therefore
> in addition

also
despite
in contrast
in conclusion
to summarize.

How many others can you think of?

▲ ... But do not join unrelated ideas

If two parts of a sentence are connected by a 'joining' word such as 'and' or 'but', make sure that there is really a logical connection between them.

In this sentence, 'and' has been used inappropriately to join two ideas:

'Asthma is an inflammatory condition of the airways and is more common in boys than girls.'

It would be better to write two separate sentences, even though both would be quite short:

'Asthma is an inflammatory condition of the airways. It is more common in boys than girls.'

▲ Construct your sentences carefully to avoid confusion ...

If you stick to the 'short sentences' and 'one idea per sentence' rule, you are less likely to end up with odd sentences like this one:

'Inhaled corticosteroids are widely used in the treatment of inflammatory disorders, including asthma, and may also be administered by the oral route, though this may be associated with a greater risk of side-effects.'

The indiscriminate use of 'and' in this sentence results in the implication that *inhaled* corticosteroids can be given by the oral route, which is clearly not what the writer intended – he meant to say 'Corticosteroids can also be administered by the oral route ...'.

However, even short sentences can be confusing (or amusing) if not carefully constructed, as in 'We treated the patients using anticholinergics'. We do not know if the writer means 'We treated those patients who used anticholinergics' or 'We treated the patients with anticholinergics'. 'I have discussed the question of feeding the rats with Professor Smith.' (Most labs prefer a more conventional diet.)

▲ Put the most important words or phrases near the beginning of the sentence

Studies of reading behaviour show that readers' attention peaks at the beginning of a sentence, with another, usually smaller, peak near the end. So it pays to put the key words or phrases near the beginning of the sentence. To illustrate this, ask yourself which of these two sentences you find easier to understand.

'To be successful, a new drug must not only be discovered, but thoroughly tested.'
'A new drug must not only be discovered, but thoroughly tested, to be successful.'

Most people find the first example easier, because it gives them a clue where they are going, rather than taking them on a 'mystery tour'.

▲ Use the active voice where appropriate …

Greater use of the active voice is a simple strategy to make your writing simpler and clearer. If you have not encountered the idea of active versus passive voice before, this is what it means. When the active voice is used, the subject of the sentence performs an action. In other words, the subject is the 'doer'.
   Here are some examples of the use of the active voice:

> Sir James Black [subject] received [verb] the Nobel Prize [object]
> Aspirin [subject] reduces [verb] inflammation [object]

When the passive voice is used, on the other hand, the object goes at the beginning of the sentence and is acted upon.

> The Nobel Prize [object] was received [verb] by Sir James Black [subject]
> Inflammation [object] is reduced [verb] by aspirin [subject]

You will notice two things about the passive voice.

1 It uses more words to say the same thing.
2 It often sounds duller.

Preferring the active voice also ties in with the idea that the most important words or phrases in a sentence should go near the beginning – provided the subject is at least as important as, or more important than, the object.

▲ ... But use the passive voice when you want to stress the object

There are three situations in which it is better to stress the object by putting it first:

1 *When the subject is unknown or unimportant.* It would be silly to say 'Some builders built the laboratory in 1991'. You would just say 'The laboratory was built in 1991'.
2 *When you want to emphasize the object.* You might want to say 'This unique process has been patented' rather than 'We have patented this unique process'.
3 *If you would rather not say who performed the action.* 'The dose was miscalculated.' Let us hope that you have no need of this last example!

▲ You can use the active voice while still remaining formal and impersonal

Some people object that you cannot use the active voice in formal writing about science, because scientific writing must be impersonal. This is a misconception. As the example 'Aspirin reduces inflammation' shows, you can use the active voice without using a person's name or personal pronoun ('I' or 'we'). In fact, nowadays, there is no reason why you should not use 'we' in formal science writing.

▲ Use parallel structures

Within sentences, you can use parallel structures to make your writing clearer. A parallel structure is a series of word groups with the same kind of structure. Using parallel structures reflects logical thinking, and helps satisfy the reader's need to see order in your writing. For example, while it is grammatically correct to say:

'This educational programme will encourage people to eat healthily, drink a sensible amount and take regular exercise.'

you might prefer to try a more elegant version of the sentence with parallel structure:

'This educational programme will encourage people to eat healthily, drink sensibly and exercise regularly.'

My favourite example of a parallel structure comes from the pen of Francis Bacon, and seems particularly appropriate for scientific writers:

'Reading maketh a full man; conference a ready man; and writing an exact man.'

(My thanks to Martin Mackay for first introducing me to this quote.)

25

Clear writing: words

Clear writing depends on selecting the right words to get your message across, precisely and economically. You need to choose words that say exactly what you mean, without taking up unnecessary space.

▲ Use simple everyday words for simple everyday things

Studies of reading difficulty show that, even for educated readers, short, familiar words make writing easier to understand. The more long, multi-syllable words a sentence contains, the harder it is to understand. So, if you want to be clear, prefer short, simple words for simple everyday things. Now, this does not mean that you cannot use scientific language. You need specific scientific terms to make your writing precise. But it does mean that you should be extra careful with your non-scientific language. Why say 'It is evident that there is a discrepancy of considerable magnitude …' when you can say 'It is clear that there is a large difference …'.

▲ Try these simple alternatives

The following list gives some examples of common long words and their shorter alternatives. None of these words is 'wrong'- in fact they can add some variety to your writing. However, (but) if you use the shorter words, say, half the time, you will have taken an important step towards clearer writing.

Instead of: *Why not use*:
purchase or acquire   buy
quantify   measure

Instead of:	*Why not use*:
communicate	write/speak
following	after
permit	let
however	but
utilize	use
manufacture	make
sufficient	enough
demonstrate	show
necessity	need
advantageous	helpful
concerning	about
discontinue	stop
endeavour	try
evident	clear
location	place
magnitude	size
participate	take part
regarding	about
remainder	rest
request	ask
requirement	need
subsequent	next

▲ Cut out unnecessary words

Even worse than the 'long words habit' is the 'wordy phrases habit'. Unlike long words, which sometimes have their place, wordy phrases are seldom justified. They make you seem pompous, and obscure your message. Here are a few of the commonest examples. If this is one of your writing problems, make your own list of 'favourite phrases' and ruthlessly eradicate them when you edit your own work.

Avoid:	*And use*:
as a means of	to
ask the question	ask
at the present time	now
during the time that	while
in order that	so that
with regard to	about
prior to	before
with the exception of	except for
a considerable number of	many

Avoid:	*And use*:
at a rapid rate	rapidly/quickly
a certain amount of	some
for the reason that	because
referred to as	called
at an early date	soon
in view of the fact that	because
during the course of	during/while

▲ Watch out for 'smothered' verbs

A 'smothered' verb is a particular kind of wordy phrase. A verb is 'smothered' when we take a perfectly good verb and make it into a noun by adding another verb, like 'make', 'take', 'give' and so on. Some examples are given in the list below. Usually, we can restore the original verb with no loss of meaning. Why not 'decide' (not 'come to a decision') to eradicate them from your writing.

Instead of:	*Use*:
make a decision	decide
come to the realization	realize
take into consideration	consider
make an estimate	estimate
give an explanation of	explain
make a presentation of	present
is indicative of	indicates
place an emphasis on	emphasize
come to a conclusion	conclude
undertake an investigation	investigate
give a description of	describe

▲ Avoid redundancy

There are some wordy phrases that you should never use, because they say the same thing twice. There is no point in saying the difference was 'large in magnitude' (or even 'large in size'). It was large, that is all you need to say. Here is a list of some common redundant phrases.

Instead of:	*Use*:
absolutely complete	complete
completely finished	finished
try and endeavour	try
meet with	meet
true facts	facts

Instead of:	*Use:*
advance plan	plan
basic essentials	basics *or* essentials
current status	status
estimate approximately	estimate
past history	history
large in size	large
few in number	few

▲ Do not be so concise that you lose the linking words and phrases

Linking words and phrases make your writing clearer by showing the connections between words, phrases, sentences and paragraphs. Examples include:

- *When you add one point to another*: and, in addition, moreover, furthermore
- *When indicating similarity*: likewise, similarly, in the same way
- *When contrasting*: but, in contrast, however, on the contrary, on the other hand, nevertheless, although, even so, in spite of/despite
- *When showing how one thing results from another*: so, therefore, hence, thus, as a result, consequently, accordingly
- *When summing up*: in conclusion, in summary, to summarize, to conclude, in brief, in other words.

▲ Use the precise word for what you mean

Be careful when choosing among scientific terms, and try to use the most specific term possible. 'Quantify,' for example, is vague. Did you 'measure', 'count', 'estimate' or 'calculate' it?

▲ Watch out for common errors of meaning

If you do not know what a word means, it is a bad idea to use it. The trouble is, some words are so commonly misused, or confused with similar-sounding words, that we *think* we know what they mean, and misuse them unknowingly. Here are some commonly confused pairs:

abrogate	abdicate
repeal or cancel out	*decline to take responsibility*
affect	effect
verb: to act upon; noun (in psychiatry): outward appearance of emotion	*verb: to bring about; noun: outcome*

alternately
every other

alternatively
offering a choice

appraise
form a judgement

apprise
inform someone

compliment
to praise something

complement
to mutually complete or add value

continual
happening over and over again

continuous
happening without interruption

definitive
stands as a definition of something

definite
precise

disinterested
unbiased by personal advantage

uninterested
does not find the subject interesting

dose
quantity administered at one time

dosage
quantity administered per unit time

infer
draw a conclusion

imply
give a hint

mitigate
make less serious or severe

militate
argue against

oral
spoken word only

verbal
spoken or written word

practical
workable, effective

practicable
feasible, i.e. capable of being done

principle
a rule

principal
the most important thing; the head of an educational institution

regime
a system of government

regimen
a system of therapy

refute
prove falsity

repudiate
claim falsity, deny

26

Clear writing: paragraphs, headings and lists

Paragraphs, headings and lists are part of the 'route map' that allows readers to find their way around your document. Once you have a clear structure in your mind (as described in Chapter 5), you need to make that structure clear to the reader by laying it out on paper.

Here are some tips to help you do this.

▲ Break up long documents with headings ...

In a scientific paper, the main headings will be dictated by the IMRAD structure (introduction, methods, results and discussion). In other kinds of scientific writing (e.g. review articles) you will have a more-or-less free hand with the headings, so do not be afraid to use them generously to help readers find their way around the document.

▲ ... And subheadings

Under your main headings, you can use subheadings. These are appropriate in most kinds of scientific writing – even in letters or memos. In original research papers, most journals will let you use subheadings within the main sections. They can be very helpful to readers, especially within long methods and results sections. You may be able to match up the methods subheadings with the results subheadings.

▲ But do not use too many levels of heading

It may be tempting, especially in a long and complex document, to use multiple levels of heading – right down to sub-sub-sub-subheadings. But this can be confusing for the reader – not to mention the writer. Usually, three levels of heading will be enough – the title or chapter heading, section headings and subheadings. If you really feel you need additional levels of headings, do not forget that you can use bulleted lists, and emboldened keywords at the beginning of sentences.

▲ Only use numbered headings if there is a good reason

Some types of document, for example, a thesis or a drug regulatory report, may have a statutory requirement for numbered headings (1.0. 1.4, 1.3.8 and so on). If so, you must comply. However, when considering introducing numbered headings into other types of document (e.g. a book or manual), ask yourself if they are really needed. Are you going to have cross-references from one section to another? Are you going to refer to the numbered sections in the index? If readers do not need the numbers to navigate the document, do not put them in. You will only be making extra work for yourself when you add new sections. If you do decide to use numbered headings, your word processor will probably be able to number and cross-reference them for you automatically (see Chapter 30).

▲ Match the style of your headings to the tone of the document

Formal scientific papers and reports will require formal headings – 'Methods,' 'Results' and so on. Subheadings will need to be brief and objective, e.g. 'Animal studies', 'Pharmacokinetics'. In other kinds of scientific writing, e.g. a magazine article, you may decide to use main headings or subheadings that actually summarize what is in the text, e.g. 'Colon cancer – the silent killer' or 'Six simple ways to cut computer costs'. In very informal writing, particularly news articles or press releases, you may decide to use headings simply to attract attention, e.g. '"It's a jungle out there," says Professor Smith'.

▲ Use plenty of paragraphs

Paragraphs are used to:

- group related thoughts
- provide visual relief.

Too many scientific papers are so mean in their use of paragraphs that you cannot see where one group of thoughts stops and the next one begins. There is no good reason for this – when you start a new topic, you should always start a new paragraph.

▲ Do not be afraid of short paragraphs

If your paragraph includes more than five to seven sentences, ask yourself whether it contains more than one group of ideas. The chances are that it does. Could it be more effectively split into two? Do not worry if you end up with two- or three-sentence paragraphs. There is nothing wrong with short paragraphs – not every train of thought can be extended into several sentences.

▲ One-sentence paragraphs are not wrong – but use them sparingly

Contrary to what you may have been taught at school, there is nothing grammatically wrong with a one-sentence paragraph. If you have only one thing to say on a particular topic, you can say it in a one-sentence paragraph.

But such paragraphs do draw attention to themselves.

So you should use one-sentence paragraphs only occasionally, for ideas that deserve emphasis. For example, the last paragraph of your paper might be a one-sentence conclusion, if that is all you have to say. One-sentence paragraphs are also useful for lists and instructions, where you want every point to stand out clearly and carry equal weight. However, if your one-sentence paragraph contains only a minor idea, you might like to merge it with an adjacent paragraph.

▲ Use topic sentences to introduce paragraphs

It is very helpful to readers if the first sentence in the paragraph gives some idea of where the paragraph is going. For example, you might say:

'Wound healing consists of three distinct phases. [topic sentence] First, an acute inflammatory phase occurs. Next, collagen synthesis repairs the wound. Finally, remodelling restores the skin's structural integrity.'

As you can see, starting with 'the bottom line' is much more effective than writing the paragraph the other way round:

'Wounding is followed by an acute inflammatory phase. Next, collagen synthesis repairs the wound. Finally, remodelling processes restore the skin's structural integrity. Thus, there are three phases to wound healing.'

▲ Use lists wherever they help readers and are allowed by the journal

In formal journal articles you may be able to use numbered lists. For example, you could list the steps in a procedure. In some journals, and in less formal scientific writing (for example a magazine article), you may also be able to use bullet-point lists. For example, the *Lancet* uses bullet-point lists of key points in articles. I have used lots of bullet-point lists in this book.

▲ Arrange items in lists in logical order

When you give a list, readers will assume that there is some logic in its order. If you list items in random order you will be confusing the reader. So think carefully about the order of items in your list. Often, the best way is to list items in order of importance, or you may want to list them in chronological or hierarchical order.

▲ Use parallel structure in lists where appropriate

If each item in the list contains several kinds of information it is appropriate to arrange them in the same order each time. A parallel structure of this kind will help readers to find their way around the list. For example:

'Wound healing consists of three phases:

1 *The acute inflammatory phase* occurs over the first few days. Neutrophils and macrophages migrate into the wound.
2 *The collagen synthesis phase* lasts for several weeks. Fibroblasts from the surrounding dermis migrate into the wound, synthesizing new collagen.
3 *The modelling phase* lasts many months. Collagen cross-linking, collagenolysis and collagen synthesis occur simultaneously, strengthening the wound.'

▲ Be consistent about capitals and full stops in lists

Different publications have their own formats for lists. In draft manuscripts and internal documents, the important thing is to be consistent about the use of capitals and full stops. The usual rule is:

• For list items that are full sentences, begin with a capital letter and end with a full stop.

- For list items that are not full sentences, but a word or phrase, begin with a lower case letter and do not use a full stop, except for the last item in the list. It is as if the list was a sentence with a full stop at the end.

For example:

'There may be various reasons why PhD theses are not submitted on time.

- The research is not complete.
- Problems may occur with data analysis.
- Writing may go more slowly than expected.
- The student may have started work on another project.'

Or:

'PhD theses may not be submitted on time because of:

- incomplete research
- problems with data analysis
- slowness in writing
- conflicting work commitments.'

27

Correct writing: common errors of grammar and idiom

The first duty of a scientific writer is to write clearly, concisely and accurately. You are not necessarily expected to be an expert on English, especially if it is not your first language. If you are submitting your work to a journal or book publisher, it will be checked carefully by a sub-editor to make sure that there are no mistakes of English grammar, idiom or spelling. The important thing is to make sure your meaning is clear, so that the sub-editor does not inadvertently misrepresent what you have to say. Note, however, that theses, conference abstracts, study reports and many other types of document are not sub-edited, so there will be no second chance to correct your mistakes before your work reaches the wider scientific community.

▲ You do not have to be an expert

This book is not a textbook of correct English. Moreover, it recognizes that most readers will be far too busy with scientific matters to spend much time perfecting their knowledge of grammar and idiom. But, bearing in mind the negative effect poor English can create, I do urge you to try to avoid unnecessary mistakes. In practical terms this means that if you are not confident in your use of English, you should get an expert to check your work before you submit it to an editor or examiner. A careful reading by a native speaker with excellent grammatical knowledge can save many embarrassing errors – this person need not necessarily be a scientific expert.

▲ Fewer allowances will be made for native English speakers

Theoretically, reviewers, thesis examiners and conference organizers should not be influenced by small mistakes in English – their job is to comment on the science. However, even trivial mistakes can be distracting, especially if they lead to confusion in meaning. Reviewers will usually make more allowances for writers for whom English is a second language than they will for native speakers. If English is your mother tongue, it may seem merely careless not to use it correctly.

▲ Find your own 'blind spots'

Many of us have just a few 'blind spots' which prevent us from producing correct copy. If so, some of the common errors listed below may help you perfect your English and make a better impression on colleagues and reviewers. Identify those that apply to you and try to memorize the correct usage.

▲ Use 'compare with' when looking for differences …

Use 'compare with' when you are looking for differences between things. Since science is so often based on looking for differences between experimental and control groups, 'compare with' is almost always correct.

Correct: 'We compared grottomycin with scabicillin.'
Incorrect: 'We compared grottomycin to scabicillin.'

▲ … And 'compare to' when you are likening one thing to another…

Occasionally, you may want to say something is like something else, in which case you use 'compared to', e.g. 'Shall I compare thee to a summer's day?'; 'The heart may be compared to a pump'.

▲ … But do not use 'compared with' where you can use 'than'

Avoid the misuse of 'compared with' as in this example.

Incorrect: 'We found a higher recovery rate in the treatment group compared with the control group.'

Correct: 'We found a higher recovery rate in the treatment group than in the control group.'

▲ Prefer 'different from'

- 'Different from ...' is the modern way.
- 'Different to ...' is the old-fashioned form, which has more or less died out.
- 'Different than ...' is acceptable only in the USA.

▲ Use 'fewer' when referring to countable nouns ...

Correct: 'Fewer psychiatric beds are needed since the introduction of care in the community' (because you could, at least in theory, count the beds).
Incorrect: 'Less psychiatric beds are needed since the introduction of care in the community.'

▲ ... But 'less' when you are referring to things that are not measured in numbers

Correct: 'There is less need for psychiatric beds since the introduction of care in the community' (because you cannot count 'need').

Oddly enough, people often use 'less' where they should use 'fewer', but they hardly ever use 'fewer' when they should use 'less'. You would never write:

Incorrect: 'There is fewer need for psychiatric beds since the introduction of care in the community.'

▲ Use 'which' for a commenting clause ...

'Which' is used in a 'commenting' or 'parenthetical' clause. If there are a pair of commas, or a pair of brackets, it is a fair bet that you should be using 'which'.

'The Thames, which flows through London, is England's largest river.'

You could take out the material starting with 'which', and the sentence would still be true. The 'which flows through London' is just giving you some extra, non-essential information.

Similarly, you would say: 'The method, which is described in detail in Appendix 1, was developed by Professor Smith.' Again, if you take out 'which is described in detail in Appendix 1', the sentence still retains the original meaning.

▲ ... And 'that' for a defining clause

'That' is used in a 'defining' clause (i.e. before a clause that could not be taken out without destroying the meaning of the sentence).

'The Thames that flows through London is heavily polluted.'

Notice, no commas, and the material after the 'that' is essential if we are to make sense of the sentence.

Similarly, you would say: 'The method that Green and White used in their first study was first described by Smith in 1996.'

▲ Watch out for verbless sentences ...

Normally, sentences must have a verb.

Incorrect: 'All good scientific papers have certain qualities in common. Such as clarity, accuracy and conciseness.'
Correct: 'All good scientific papers have certain qualities in common, such as clarity, accuracy and conciseness.'
Also correct: 'All good scientific papers have certain qualities in common. These include clarity, accuracy and conciseness.'

▲ ... But you can miss out verbs when writing notes, or in items in lists

You can, however, miss out verbs when you are writing in note form, or in items in lists.

'All good scientific papers have certain qualities in common:

• clear sentences
• accurate word choice
• concise construction.'

Verbless sentences are sometimes also used in informal writing for dramatic effect. You may be able to spot one or two in this book. Like this one.

▲ Watch out for mixed singular and plural verbs and nouns

'The solutions was mixed ...' is obviously wrong. Other singular/plural problems are more difficult to spot.

Incorrect: 'Each of our lecturers have a postgraduate degree.'
Correct: 'Each of our lecturers has a postgraduate degree' (because you are referring to each lecturer, not the lecturers as a group).
But: 'All our lecturers have postgraduate degrees' (because you are referring to all the lecturers).

▲ Remember that companies are singular

Singular verbs are used with the names of companies, thus:

Incorrect: 'Megapharm are developing bradykinin antagonists.'
Correct: 'Megapharm is developing bradykinin antagonists.'

▲ Use apostrophes carefully in possessives

Put the apostrophe before the 's' when you are talking about something belonging to just one thing, or to a person, e.g. 'The university's records' (belonging to just one university); 'Professor Smith's experiment' (belonging to Professor Smith). But put it after the 's' when you are talking about something belonging to more than one thing, e.g. 'The universities' records' (more than one university).

▲ Remember that there are special rules for 'it'

The exception to the rule above is the apostrophe used with 'it'. 'It's' is short for 'it is', e.g. 'It's usually warm in summer' (i.e. the abbreviated form of it is). 'Its' for 'belonging to it' has no apostrophe, e.g. 'The reading was twice its usual value' (belonging to it).

▲ There are no apostrophes in plurals

There is no place for the apostrophe when you are simply using the 's' to denote a plural.

Incorrect: 'Supervisor's should help their students.'
Correct: 'Supervisors should help their students.'

▲ Avoid contractions such as 'it's' and 'don't' in formal science writing

In informal writing or reported speech, an apostrophe can be used to replace a missing letter, as in 'don't' (short for 'do not') and 'here's' (short for 'here is'). However, it is better to avoid them in formal science writing.

▲ Split infinitives only if there is no better way of writing the sentence

Split infinitives are widely regarded as an error in UK English, though they are not considered so in US English. 'Split infinitive' means putting an adjective or adverb between 'to' and the infinitive form of the verb. The classic example is from Star Trek: 'To boldly go where no man has gone before.'

Another example: 'It is essential to fully evaluate all the programs before making a decision.'

The non-split version would be: 'It is essential to evaluate all the programs fully before making a decision.'

Any UK grammar textbook will tell you that splitting an infinitive is not a true grammatical error, but that it is very widely disliked. To avoid annoyance, do not use split infinitives. However, split rather than write an ugly sentence.

▲ Beware 'false' split infinitives

Note that, contrary to what some people imagine, the following example does not contain a split infinitive, because 'we' are doing the evaluating. The infinitive 'to evaluate' is not used, and therefore there is nothing to split: 'We will fully evaluate all the programs before making a decision.'

28

Overcoming writer's block

Have you ever spent hours staring at a blank screen or piece of paper, unable to get started? This phenomenon is known as writer's block. We all experience it once in a while, but for some people it becomes a frequent problem, reducing their writing productivity.

Everyone has their own way of beating writer's block, and the list of tips below is made up of helpful suggestions from many sufferers. Among these ideas, you may find the right one to help you.

▲ Plan carefully

It is impossible to overemphasize the importance of planning. Meticulous preparation not only determines the quality of the finished product, it also affects your psychological approach to writing. If you have planned the whole of your project in advance, and broken it down into manageable chunks, you will:

- know what you are going to say in each section
- have confidence in your ability to complete it on time
- be able to start anywhere in the project, as convenient.

▲ Start with the easy bits

It will help to build your confidence, and speed up your writing, if you start wherever seems easiest. You can do this if you have a good plan. Often, in an original research paper, the methods and results sections are the easiest places to start. You may well already have a written protocol for the methods. For the results, there will be relatively little choice about what you have to say, and again you will already have it written down in your lab book or a study report.

▲ Go with the flow

Perhaps the most important advice is 'If it ain't broke, don't fix it'. If your work is going well, and the writing flows in a continuous stream, do not stop until you begin to run out of energy or enthusiasm. When you do begin to flag, take a break (see below).

▲ Take a break when you feel you need one …

You may need quite frequent breaks when concentrating hard – a ten-minute break every hour, or even every half-hour, is not too much. Taking a short break will not disrupt your concentration – in fact, it will help you to focus on the task in hand.

▲ … But not for too long

Studies show that short breaks are the most effective in aiding concentration. Long breaks (say 20 minutes or more) do not provide any additional benefit, and may simply indicate that you are procrastinating.

▲ Get away from it during breaks

When you take a break, do not just sit there – move around, go and talk to someone, or get some fresh air or exercise – you might even want to use your ten minutes to take a brisk walk, indoors or out, or even ride an exercise bike or do some exercises in your office.

▲ Sleep on it if stuck

If you are stuck, and a short break does not help, it may be time to stop and do something else. Sleep on the problem, and in the morning you may come back to it with fresh ideas and enthusiasm.

▲ Talk to someone

It may help to ask a colleague for help. Even simply talking about the problem to someone else, without looking for any particular advice, may be beneficial. Often, an 'outsider' will be able to provide a fresh viewpoint that gives you the impetus you need to get going again.

▲ Write a 'letter to Auntie'

If you are stuck trying to explain a complex concept, it can be helpful to imagine that you are writing to a non-expert about the topic. You might choose a favourite aunt, who is very interested in everything you do, but is not scientifically qualified. If you can explain your point to an interested lay person, you can be sure that you will have expressed yourself clearly. Then all you have to do is reintroduce the scientific terminology into your clear explanation, and you have suddenly solved your problem.

▲ Read around the subject

Sometimes, you can get a fresh perspective by reading about the topic. There is nothing wrong with looking at how other writers have tackled the same problem. You can borrow ideas and approaches without using the same words.

▲ Clear your desk

If other projects are cluttering up your desk you will have two problems:

1 you won't be able to find all the papers you need for your current project
2 the clutter will distract you – it too is waiting for attention.

So, clear your desk of everything except the project in hand. If you have an in-tray, put it behind you, or in a cupboard, out of sight.

▲ Think positively

This book is based on the belief that all scientists can learn how to write. Some of us may have more natural talent than others but, with a little encouragement and tuition, *everyone* can do it reasonably well. If, due to negative past experiences, voices tend to play in your head saying 'I'm no good at this' or 'I'll never be able do it in the time I have left', try to replace them with positive thoughts. Think: 'I can do this, I just have to complete all the sections of my plan' or 'You only have to finish one section today'.

▲ Do not try to get everything right first time

You can get hopelessly stuck and dispirited if you keep going over and over the same sentence, trying unsuccessfully to get it just right. For most people, it is better to try to get something down for every section, even if you know it is far from perfect. Then you can go back and revise – having completed the first draft quickly, you will have plenty of time for revisions.

▲ If stuck, just write

A standard technique for overcoming writer's block involves simply writing the first thing that comes into your head, however ludicrous. The important thing is that it gets you started on the physical process of writing. You will soon find that your random musings turn into comprehensible thoughts about the subject in hand.

▲ Write around missing information

If, in the middle of writing, you find that you do not have all the facts or references you need, do not waste time thinking or worrying about it, or break your concentration to go looking for them. Make a note to yourself in the manuscript about the missing information. You can use the hidden text feature of your word processor to do this. Then you can save your queries up to be answered in a single trip to the library or on-line session.

▲ Do not stop when you are winning

Even when you come to the end of a section, do not automatically stop. Sometimes it helps to get down the first few sentences of the next section. That way, when you come back to it the next day, you will have the confidence-building feeling of having already made a start on the next task.

▲ Set crazy deadlines ...

In Chapter 29, we will talk about setting real-life deadlines for your project. However, if you have writer's block, it can also help to set yourself crazy, short-term deadlines. For example, you may say to yourself 'I have to get 200 words written by 3 o'clock'.

▲ ... And reward yourself for meeting them

You can offer yourself rewards for meeting your crazy deadlines. 'If I have written 200 words by 3 o'clock I will have a cup of coffee/go for a walk/telephone a friend.' It is tempting to offer yourself rewards in the shape of food, but this can prove unhealthy in the long term, especially if you are writing a large thesis or a book!

29

Managing your time for writing and revising

Writing can be a time-consuming process. Many scientific and technical professionals feel overwhelmed by the amount of time needed to write 'essential' documents such as papers, theses, reports and grant proposals – not to mention 'optional' tasks such as reviews, book chapters and magazine articles.

Yet, writing is so essential to a successful scientific career that we simply must find ways of doing it efficiently. Here are some tips that will help you to make the most of your writing time, and feel better about your productivity.

▲ Remember the 'one-third rule'

For major writing projects, a good rule of thumb is 'one-third planning, one third writing, one-third revising'. It may seem daunting to spend so much time on planning your work, but it will pay dividends. When you do sit down to write, you will be so confident of what you want to say that progress will be very fast. At first glance, you may also think that a third of your time spent revising is too much. Realistically, however, you are unlikely to produce your best work without spending a considerable time revising your first draft.

▲ Draw up a writing schedule

For a big project, it will help to divide the work up into manageable chunks, and set interim deadlines. When you draw up your writing schedule, remember to include time to:

- obtain references
- plan the project

- write the first draft
- revise the first draft
- circulate the manuscript to your colleagues or boss
- incorporate comments into a second draft
- prepare figures, photographs and any other illustrative materials
- obtain any necessary final approvals or sign-offs.

▲ Break your work down into manageable chunks

'An elephant is easier to eat if you slice it first.' A 50 000 word thesis seems like a terrifying amount. However, it is only 200 words a day for a year (excluding weekends, of course). Or, if you start very late, it is 2000 words a day for a month. Both would be perfectly manageable – all you need is motivation and organization.

▲ Block out writing time in your diary

Writing time is just as important as research time or meetings time. The danger is that it will be squeezed out by other duties. While some of us do find time to write in the minutes in between appointments, many people find that they need to write in chunks of at least an hour, especially when writing the first draft. It takes time to remember where you left off, and what you want to say next. Blocking time out in your diary shows that you take your writing commitments seriously.

▲ Make sure your colleagues are organized too

If you are writing a paper with co-authors (see below), make sure that everyone books writing and revising time into their diaries. Otherwise, you may find that just when you need a colleague's advice or input on a particular section, he or she is too busy or away at a conference.

▲ When writing as part of a team, define responsibilities

If several people are to take part in writing a document, make sure that the responsibilities of each member of the group are clearly defined. If you want people to actually write particular sections, make sure they know exactly what is required in terms of content and length. If you want people to comment, make it clear (preferably in a note attached to the typescript) whether you want advice on the scientific content, the writing style, spelling and grammar, or all of these.

▲ Be realistic about how fast you write

It may help to time-check how many words you can write in an average hour or day. We all have our different ways of writing, and some individuals are more productive than others. While it is possible to improve your productivity by writing more efficiently, as outlined in Chapter 5, it is also important to be realistic. Even when things are going well, and you have no distractions or other commitments, you are unlikely to be able to write more than a couple of thousand words of carefully considered prose in a day. Trying to write a 10 000-word dissertation overnight is just not going to be feasible.

▲ Make sure you have the right tools for the job

Writing is likely to go much faster if you have the right tools, such as:

• references and background materials
• dictionaries, abbreviations lists and other reference books
• reference management program (see Chapter 31)
• software for drawing graphs and diagrams.

If you work in a company or academic institution, it is worth persuading your department to invest in the best tools it can afford, so that you can write more efficiently and have more time to get on with the rest of your work.

▲ Use spare moments for non-creative tasks

You may need peace and quiet and time to think in order to write your best prose. However, you may not need such 'quality time' to perform more mundane tasks, such as revising your work or typing references into your reference management database. Make yourself a list of tasks you can accomplish when you have a spare ten minutes.

▲ Make use of travelling time

In today's busy world, often the only time we get to be alone and think is on a long journey, by train or by plane. This can be good writing or revising time. Try taking a manuscript with you to revise. Or take your lap-top or palm-top computer with you. Make sure you have extra batteries to allow you to work for several hours on a long journey.

▲ Do not waste time looking for things

All writers should recognize that the average person can spend up to half an hour each day just looking for the documents or other items needed to do their work. Have an efficient filing system for your references, notes and other documents. Make sure that each draft is dated so that you can distinguish between multiple copies of your latest writing project. Some word processors will automatically insert a date in a 'footer'. What applies to your filing cabinet also applies to the hard disk of your computer – make sure that you put all the files relating to a particular project in a logical place – one folder (directory) per project is a good general rule.

30

Using your word processor more effectively

Nowadays most of us will be writing using a word-processing program. This has undoubtedly made writing much easier for most people. It seems amazing that when word processors were first introduced, there were dire warnings that the standards of writing would drop. On the contrary, standards of writing and presentation have improved. Because it is so easy to make corrections, and to move text around using a word processor, scientists' manuscripts are probably more polished than ever before.

▲ Build up a personal list of hints

The tips in this section will get you started. You will undoubtedly discover many more from colleagues, articles in computer magazines and manuals, and online. Do not confine yourself to the manuals that came with the program – published books such as the *Idiot's Guide* and *... for Dummies* series are often more informative and user-friendly.

▲ Get to know your own word processor

A little time spent practising and experimenting with your word processor will pay long-term dividends, by making your writing more efficient and freeing you to concentrate on other tasks. The tips given here apply to most of the commonly used word processors, such as Word or WordPerfect. If you use a different program, check your manual or on-line help to see whether your word processor offers these features.

▲ Programme your word processor to finish complicated words

Many word processors have a function whereby you can automatically finish certain words or phrases. For example, you could programme the word processor so that every time you type 'fluv …' it will finish the word as 'fluvoxamine'. However, this only works if the first few letters are unique to your chosen word. A better technique for words beginning with common letters would be to be programme short-cut keys (see below).

▲ Programme short-cut keys for complicated words and phrases

You can programme your own short-cut keys so that you can easily insert long or difficult-to-type phrases such as 'α_2-adrenergic agonist' by just typing, for example, 'Alt-X'.

▲ Learn your word processor's short-cut keys for frequently used symbols

If you have to use Greek characters or mathematical symbols frequently, it will pay you to learn the relevant short-cut keys, rather than selecting characters from a menu. If there is no key-stroke short cut for the character you want, you can create one (see above).

▲ Use the right spell checker

If you are writing for a US publication, use the US English spell checker. Use the UK English spell checker for a UK publication. In UK English, some words can have more than one correct spelling, such as 'randomise' or 'randomize'. In such instances, be consistent, and adjust your spell-checker dictionary accordingly.

▲ Customize your dictionary

When you use a technical word that your spell checker does not recognize, add it to your dictionary. That way, it will recognize the word in the future.

▲ Use your grammar checker selectively

Grammar checkers are useful under some circumstances – for example, you may find it helpful to calculate the readability index of your writing, or percentage of active versus passive voice. However, grammar checkers are no substitute for careful reading by a native speaker. They do not pick up all mistakes, and sometimes indicate a mistake where none exists. They are also frustratingly slow.

▲ Customize your tool bar (in Windows programs)

You can customize your tool bar so that functions you use frequently can be accessed quickly and easily, while functions you never use can be hidden away.

▲ Get to know the tables function

The tables function included in the more sophisticated word processors, such as Word or WordPerfect, can save you hours of time. Not only can you format tables in a wide range of styles, you can also use tables as mini-spreadsheets. Check the journal's Instructions to Authors regarding the formatting of tables.

▲ Get a fresh view

Changing the way in which you view your document may help you to write more effectively. For example, even if you are writing a manuscript that must be double spaced, you may prefer to work on it single spaced, so that you can see more of the text. Double spacing can then be specified at a late stage, when you are happy with the rest of the document. When polishing your document, viewing it in whole-page mode (also known as print preview) will enable you to detect problems such as headings that appear on the last line of the page, with their associated text on the next page.

▲ Use hidden text to write notes to yourself

When writing your first draft, you may want to insert notes and queries to remind you to address certain issues later. You can insert these as hidden text, so that you can print off clean copies for others to see. Do not forget to remove the hidden text at a later date. If you are submitting the document to a journal electronically, hidden text may confuse its desktop publishing systems.

▲ Use automatic formatting features ... cautiously

You can automatically format headings, subheadings, sub-subheadings and so on. This is particularly useful in long documents with many headings, such as a thesis. However, be aware that some journals like you to put in as little formatting as possible. This is because there may be an incompatibility between your word-processing program and their desktop publishing software. Check the Instructions to Authors to see whether headings should be underlined, emboldened or otherwise distinguished.

▲ Generate contents lists automatically

Automatic formatting also allows you to generate contents lists – again, a useful feature in long and complicated documents.

▲ Use templates for standard documents wherever possible

Some journals supply templates for papers (also available in reference management software).

▲ Be your own desktop publisher

For documents that are not going to be typeset by a journal, but simply printed in your office (for example, a thesis, report or manual) use the desktop publishing features of your word processor. This will enable you to produce smart-looking documents without having to go to the trouble of learning to use a specialist desktop publishing program. For example, Word provides a range of standard formats for reports, letters, faxes, theses and newsletters.

31

Useful software for writers

In addition to word processors, other programs and peripheral devices have also revolutionized the way we prepare scientific manuscripts. This section lists just some of the programs and peripherals I have found most helpful for writing.

▲ Reference management software

As described in Chapter 16, reference management software helps you deal with references more efficiently. This is especially important if you are writing a document with many references, such as a review article or thesis. Each reference is inserted in a database using a standard form. This way, you never have to type the same reference more than once. You do not even have to type it if you download it from PubMed or another online service. Once your references are in the database, you can simply insert them into your paper as temporary citations, and then format it according to various standard journal styles. You can programme your own styles if you need to, but the programs include so many that you will probably never need to do this. Reference management programs make light work of renumbering or reordering your references when you make changes to a document.

The commonest programs are EndNote, Reference Manager and ProCite.

Endnote
www.endnote.com

Reference Manager
www.refman.com

ProCite
www.procite.com

▲ Mind-mapping software

As described in Chapter 5, mind-mapping is a technique that will help you plan documents and presentations. It can be easier to prepare a mind map on your computer than on paper, as you can drag and drop items from one part of your mind map to another, instead of writing items then scribbling them out. Mind-mapping software also allows you to create a formal outline from your finished mind map, and to add notes to each item in the map. Commercially available programs include MindManager, MindGenius and Mindmapper, but there are many others.

MindManager
www.mindjet.com

MindGenius
www.mindgenius.com

Mindmapper
www.mindmapper.com

▲ Voice recognition software

Most of this book was written using voice recognition software. These programs have only recently become suitable for general use, but look set to have a big impact on the way we write. The programs come with an inbuilt vocabulary, to which you can add new words.

If you find typing difficult, or you make a lot of mistakes, voice recognition will help you improve your productivity. You need a computer with a sound card and speakers, plus a microphone to speak into. The programs recognize most of what you say straight out of the box, but you can improve recognition by training them. When the program fails to recognize a word you can either select a word from a list given, or type in a replacement word. The best known programs are Dragon NaturallySpeaking and IBM ViaVoice.

Dragon NaturallySpeaking
www.nuance.com

IBM ViaVoice
www.software.ibm.com/speech/

▲ Electronic medical dictionaries

The well-known *Stedman's Medical Dictionary* and *Dorland's Medical Dictionary* have given rise to a range of software products and online medical dictionaries.

Stedman's
www.stedmans.com

Dorland's
www.dorlands.com

32

Writers' resources on the World Wide Web

It would be impossible to list all the pages of interest to biomedical writers on the World Wide Web. Just a few personal favourites are listed here – most have links to other interesting resources. Many biomedical journals now publish their Instructions to Authors on the Web – use any search engine to track down the journal of your choice.

▲ Uniform Requirements for Manuscripts Submitted to Biomedical Journals

www.icmje.org

▲ Strunk & White's Elements of Style

www.bartleby.com/141/
  The well-known style guide online.

▲ American Medical Writers Association (AMWA)

http://www.amwa.org

The American Medical Writers Association (AMWA), founded in 1940, is a non-profit organization of professionals engaged in medical communications. AMWA provides a forum for the exchange of ideas and the improvement of professional writing skills. Services and activities include meetings and conferences, seminars and workshops, and a quarterly journal.

▲ European Medical Writers Association (EMWA)

www.emwa.org

The European Medical Writers Association is a chapter of the American Medical Writers Association (AMWA). As well as the benefits of belonging to AMWA, EMWA members receive a newsletter several times a year and have the opportunity to attend the EMWA conference which is held in a different European location each Spring. EMWA's membership includes academics and professionals working in-house or freelance for pharmaceutical and medical communications companies and research institutes, or in the wider field of journalism.

▲ Canada Chapter – American Medical Writers' Association

www.amwa-canada.ca

Contains many useful links.

33

Selected further reading

Listed below are some of the books I have found most useful.

▲ Biomedical writing

Albert T (2000) *Winning the Publications Game*. Radcliffe Publishing Ltd, Oxford.

Davis M (2004) *Scientific Papers and Presentations*. Academic Press, San Diego.

Day R A and Gastel B (2006) *How to Write and Publish a Scientific Paper*. Cambridge University Press, Cambridge.

Hall G M (2003) *How to Write a Paper*. BMJ Books, London.

Huth E J (1990) *How to Write and Publish Papers in the Medical Sciences*. Williams & Wilkins, Philadelphia.

Matthews J R, Bowen J M and Matthews R W (2007) *Successful Scientific Writing*. Cambridge University Press, Cambridge.

O'Connor M (1986) *How to Copyedit Scientific Books and Journals*. ISI Press, Philadelphia.

O'Connor M (1991) *Writing Successfully in Science*. Routledge, London.

Wager E, Godlee F and Jefferson T (2002) *How to Survive Peer Review*. BMJ Books, London.

Wager E (2005) *Getting Research Published: An A–Z of Publication Strategy*. Radcliffe Publishing Ltd, Oxford.

▲ Biomedical style manuals

American Medical Association (2007) *AMA Manual of Style*. Oxford University Press Inc, USA.

Council of Science Editors (2006) *Scientific Style and Format*. Council of Science Editors, Virginia, USA.

▲ Planning techniques

Buzan T (2006) *The Ultimate Book of Mind Maps*. Harper Thorsons, London.
Minto B (2001) *The Pyramid Principle*. Financial Times Prentice Hall, London.

▲ Use of English

Burchfield R W (2004) *Fowler's Modern English Usage*. Oxford University Press, Oxford.
Gowers E (1987) *The Complete Plain Words*. Penguin, London.
Strunk W and White E B (1999) *The Elements of Style*. Longman, UK.
Truss L (2005) *Eats, Shoots and Leaves: the Zero Tolerance Approach to Punctuation*. Profile Books Ltd, London.

Appendix:
Manuscript checklist

1 Is the content appropriate for the intended audience?
2 Is the structure logical and does it cover all relevant aspects?
3 Is there any superfluous material that should be edited out?
4 Is it complete? Check:

- ❏ title page, if required
- ❏ authors in correct order with initials, degrees, affiliations etc. in correct journal style
- ❏ name and address of corresponding author indicated
- ❏ contents page, if required – entries should match headings exactly
- ❏ abstract, if required
- ❏ all sections of main text
- ❏ references
- ❏ acknowledgements
- ❏ appendices
- ❏ tables
- ❏ figures
- ❏ figure legends.

5 Are pages numbered?

6 Headings

- ❏ Are first- second- and third order headings used correctly and clearly distinguished? (It often helps to write them all down on a separate sheet of paper.)
- ❏ Are they in a logical order?
- ❏ Are they consistently worded, and are capitals used consistently and according to journal or house style?
- ❏ No full stops at the end of headings.

7 Tables

- ❏ Is their layout clear and not unnecessarily complicated?
- ❏ Do they duplicate information in the text?
- ❏ Are they all referred to in the text, in correct numerical order?
- ❏ Do they show what the text says they show?
- ❏ Does the title explain what is in the table?
- ❏ Does the title follow the correct style for the journal?
- ❏ Are abbreviations explained?
- ❏ Are footnote indicators correctly used, and attached to the right footnote?
- ❏ Do totals in columns add up correctly?
- ❏ Is their approximate location indicated in the text?

8 Figures

- ❏ Do they duplicate information in the text?
- ❏ Are they all referred to in the text, in correct numerical order?
- ❏ Do they show what the text says they show?
- ❏ Does the title explain what is in the figure?
- ❏ Does the legend follow the correct style for the journal?
- ❏ Does shading or colour on keys correspond to the figure?
- ❏ Are abbreviations explained?
- ❏ Are footnote indicators correctly used, and attached to the right footnote?
- ❏ Is cropping indicated on photographs?
- ❏ Is their approximate location indicated in the text?

9 References

- ❏ Are all references cited in the text in the reference list and vice versa?
- ❏ Do numbered references refer to the right reference?
- ❏ Does each reference contain all the necessary elements?
- ❏ Are they cited in the correct style?
- ❏ Are standard journal abbreviations used (*Index Medicus*)?

10 Are cross-references to other chapters, section numbers etc. correct? Are cross-references to page numbers marked for completion after typesetting?

11 Abbreviations

- ❏ Only used when needed.
- ❏ SI abbreviations need not be spelt out.
- ❏ Others spelt out on first mention in the body text (not just the abstract).

12 Spelling

- ❏ English or American?
- ❏ Must read as well as running a computer spell check.
- ❏ Check names of drugs, organisms etc. carefully.

13 Grammar – watch out for:

❏ incomplete sentences
❏ dangling participles
❏ subject-verb mismatches
❏ wrong use of tenses.

14 Punctuation

❏ Brackets and quotation marks – do they come in pairs?
❏ Are commas, semicolons etc. correctly used?

Index